The "Ah Ha's" of Weight Loss

A Common Sense Approach to Fitness & Nutrition

Brad LaTour

The "Ah Ha's" of Weight Loss — A Common Sense Approach to Fitness & Nutrition

Copyright © 2009 by Brad LaTour

All rights reserved. This publication, or parts thereof, may not be reproduced in any manner whatsoever without written permission of the publisher.

Published by: Body by One
                1834 George Ave.
                Annapolis, MD 21401
                443-433-0597

Contact the author: blatour@jumpsnap.com

Edited by Cheryl Drake
Interior Design by Lisa Liddy
Cover Design by Deb Forish

Printed and Bound in the United States of America

12 11 10 09 08   5 4 3 2 1

ISBN: 978-0-615-23195-2

Dedication

I dedicate this book to you. We've likely never met, and yet you and others like you have inspired me to write this, my first book. Your commitment to losing weight and living a healthier life has led me to take on this challenge. I've finally unlocked the simple secrets of a healthier lifestyle and have pushed past the road blocks that always prevented me from achieving my goal weight, so now is the right time to share these "secrets" with you.

If you're struggling today, feeling frustrated or even hopeless about achieving your weight loss goals, I assure you that there IS a sustainable solution that will work for you. Pulling from my experiences, I promise that the common sense approach and techniques I suggest will finally allow you to get on and stay on the path toward sustainable, healthy living.

You have the power to make a change, and you control the desire to make it happen. It won't happen overnight, and it will indeed be a series of small adjustments as opposed to one magical solution. I dedicate this book to you because I believe you can be successful just as I was and continue to be.

Enjoy the book. Put yourself first for a change, and allow yourself to truly absorb each **Ah Ha** without any distractions. I'm certain many people rely on and look up to you, so make the most important commitment to them and yourself by choosing healthy living.

Healthy Jumping…

Brad LaTour
blatour@jumpsnap.com

Table of Contents

Introduction	1
About the Author	9
Ah Ha #1: Magic Pills Just Don't Exist	11
Ah Ha #2: It's Simple Math—Calories Consumed vs. Calories Burned	15
Ah Ha #3: How to Lose a Pound Mathematically	36
Ah Ha #4: Exercise, Exercise, Exercise	42
Ah Ha #5: Make Fitness a Budget Item	50
Ah Ha #6: Your Most Power Exercise Equipment: Your Brain	56
Ah Ha #7: Muscle is Your Friend	61
Ah Ha #8: Take the Stairs	64
Ah Ha #9: Fast Food isn't New—The Lack of Exercise Is	70
Ah Ha # 10: Focus on Nutrition, Not Diet	76
Ah Ha #11: Never Skip Breakfast	79
Ah Ha #12: Never Say "Never"	85
Ah Ha #13: Wasted Calories—Liquids	90
Ah Ha #14: Nutrition Labels 101	97

Ah Ha #15: Portion Control Means Gaining Control	106
Ah Ha #16: If You Don't Want to Eat It, Don't Bring it Home	111
Ah Ha #17: You Can't Reach a Goal Tomorrow if You Don't Know Where You Are Today	117
Ah Ha #18: How to Measure Success	123
Ah Ha #19: Take Lots of Pictures; They Don't Lie	127
Ah Ha #20: Never Too Late to Start	130
Ah Ha #21: Anything Worth Having Takes Hard Work and Commitment	133
Ah Ha #22: The Dreaded Annual Physical	136
Ah Ha #23: If you Really Love Them, Be Honest	139
Ah Ha #24: "Overnight Success" . . . Only in Hollywood	142
Ah Ha #25: Obesity Facts—You Can Make a Difference!	146

Acknowledgments

With the support and encouragement of others, I have been able to achieve this very special goal of writing my first book.

Thank you to my wife, Susan, and my girls, Cate and Emily. My weight loss journey began when Susan was pregnant with our first child, Cate. I remember vividly when we were only about 4 weeks pregnant and I realized that I needed to be a much stronger role model to my future child. I didn't want to miss out on any activities because I was out of shape, lethargic or simply unable to participate.

Thank you to my parents, Chas and Dian, for believing in me and reminding me about skills and talents I didn't know I had or that were collecting dust. I thank them for their endless years of sacrifice that I can more genuinely appreciate now that I have become a parent myself.

Thank you to my business partner and best friend, Mike Walden, for his years of friendship and belief in me. Our friendship dates all the way back to the 7th grade. This level of friendship paves the way for crucial, real honesty when embarking on a project as large as JumpSnap and its supporting products.

Thank you to Andy Tobias who has been my mentor throughout the entire process of developing JumpSnap. He enabled me to take an idea and transform it into a marketable product that has given me the platform to pursue other passions like writing this book.

I send a special thank you to my customers. I have built a business dedicated to putting customers first and providing the best possible products and supporting content to allow them to achieve their health and fitness goals. I am very proud of the countless emails I receive from customers sharing their success stories that inspire me every day.

Thank you to everyone who has been so supportive along the way. You know who you are, so please accept my heartfelt "thank you."

Introduction

When it comes to weight loss, fitness, and healthy living, the marketplace is inundated with marketing gimmicks and false promises. It's easy to get confused and wrapped up in all the hype, as I have been on occasion. No wonder our chances of weight loss success are stacked against us.

So how is this book any different? My approach is to lay out the facts stripped of the advertising hype and allow you to use them to your advantage. You may or may not have noticed that there is no mention of the word "diet" in the title. It candidly may hurt book sales, but it is clearly by design. If I achieve my goal, you'll read this book and reflect. You'll have a conversation with yourself that might go something like this, "I know eating that fast food burger and fries isn't good for me, but now I at least know the degree to which it is sabotaging my goals." This subtle change in mindset will help you achieve sustainable success and finally defy the enticing diet community who posts a dismal 95% FAILURE rate. The increase in obesity rates is undeniable and getting worse. If we're not ready today for a completely different approach, then I don't know when we will be.

Before you can understand my approach and fully appreciate my story of personal achievement that led me to write this book, allow me to give you some background. Growing up, I was a very active youth constantly playing outside and later participating in multiple sports like soccer, tennis, wrestling and lacrosse. I grew up in a household that ate dinner together often and did not substitute good quality food with easy-to-consume fast food.

I graduated in 1987 from Radnor High School located just outside of Philadelphia, Pennsylvania. At that point I stopped growing. That meant I graduated at an intimidating 5' 8" and 135 pounds. Yeah, I know, a little scrawny, but I was tough. I only remember these weights so vividly because I wrestled. (Wrestlers compete according to weight classes.) I also remember this weight because when I attended the great Penn State University in the summer of 1987, I put on 20 pounds of muscle. No, seriously, it was 20 pounds of muscle because it was really the first time in my life I had ever lifted weights, which I did consistently all summer long. In fact, it was probably the most my body changed in any given period of my life. I remained very active throughout my four years in Happy Valley and likely graduated around 160 to 165 pounds.

Within the first five years of graduation, I remained active and participated in triathlons (swim, bike, run), weekly softball games, and adult soccer games. I even ran in the famous Washington D.C. based Marine Corps Marathon in 1994 and 1995. At this point, I had no concern about weight gain. In fact, I didn't even start worrying about weight gain until I was 28 years old in 1997. At that point in my life, as it is for so many of us, the job became my number one priority. This isn't necessarily a bad thing, but it did come with a cost that, in retrospect, was my health.

Because I was determined to be the first at the office in the morning and the last to go home in the evening, I started making bad decisions, such as not eating breakfast, eating lunch at 2 p.m. or 3 p.m., and then eating a less-than-nutritious dinner. About that time I started asking myself, "How am I gaining weight if I'm only eating twice per day?" I asked the question, but I certainly didn't do much to change the outcome, especially since I had the job to worry about first. Sound familiar? Coincidentally, these new eating patterns couldn't have come at a worse time given the fact that my metabolism was naturally going to slow down with age anyway, so I was really compounding the problem. I did this knowingly but without any real understanding—a key distinction. Knowing something doesn't usually drive us to dig much below the surface on the topic while understanding it means we realize there is some degree of impact. Taking the knowledge gained from the understanding and applying it results in the "Ah Ha" moment that leads to lifestyle changes and sustainable success.

From 1997 through 2004 I experienced my progressive, yet subtle weight gain. I'm fortunate that I have fairly broad shoulders, so I carried it well and most people wouldn't have considered me to be overweight. I'm not so sure this is really a blessing because it probably numbed me to the inevitable that I was gaining weight. Throughout these years, I gained approximately seven to eight pounds per year until I reached my breaking point. Mind you, I got married in 2002, and like most soon-to-be spouses, I joined a health club with the intent of losing the weight before the big day. Granted I did lose maybe 10–15 pounds prior to the big day, but I was still around 180 pounds. When I look at my wedding photos now, I look huge compared to my current weight. It probably didn't help that my wife looked amazingly beautiful with her toned body and 100 pound frame.

So what changed? Why didn't I continue down the path of gradual weight gain or maintain the same unhealthy levels I had already created for myself? I took control of the situation and said, "Enough is enough." I know, earth shattering, right? Seriously though, the math of losing weight really isn't very difficult to understand; in fact, it's simple. The key, and what I hope you take away from my story, is that you need to allow yourself to absorb the fundamentals which also means to stop believing the hype. The hype I refer to is the constant barrage of pills, gels, shakes, and any number of quick fixes to weight loss. As the old saying goes, "If it sounds too good to be true, then it likely is."

"Ah Ha" Moments

What are Ah Ha moments? Surely you've experienced them many times throughout your life. They come in big and small moments when something clicks and a concept or application or process that was previously murky, becomes crystal clear. They are usually followed by a quick burst of adrenalin to mark the point of success. Sometimes, we even step back and laugh because the Ah Ha was staring us right in the face, but we needed to view it from a different angle to realize it. Sound familiar? They occur in all aspects of our lives, and they should be celebrated because they often define a small victory.

I think we all need to rejoice and appreciate more of the small victories in life we so often allow to pass us by. The real benefit of an Ah Ha is that it means you are engaged, listening to yourself and not simply going through the motions. It reflects a level of desired understanding with a bigger purpose in mind. With a topic like weight loss and sustainable healthy living, the real achievement comes when combining many individual Ah Ha moments to form sustainable healthy habits that last a lifetime.

I know exactly when I had my first incident that drove me to discover these future Ah Ha moments. It was the fall of 2004, and I was in my closet simply distraught that my size 36 inch waist pants were getting too tight. It was traumatic enough that about four years earlier I had to transition from a size 34 that I wore much of my adult life to a size 36. Now I was on the verge of having to purchase 38 inch pants. There was just no way I was going to allow that to happen.

There were two more life events that strengthened my determination. After two miscarriages, my wife was four weeks pregnant with our first daughter, Cate Marie LaTour, who would later join the world in August of 2005. As life would have it, my father-in-law, Henry Heishman, was losing his battle with cancer and would later pass away in December 2004. I remember vividly that I had to scour my closet to find a suit for the funeral that I could wear—not an easy task. I finally settled on the one that was the least uncomfortable but by no means fit well. It was also a struggle to find a dress shirt that didn't cut off the circulation in my neck. I'm actually a little embarrassed to say that I had to unbutton the top button soon after the funeral because I was so uncomfortable.

That was really the last straw. It became very clear to me that I had to take control over the one thing in my life that was getting the best of me. I had to do it for my unborn child so that I could lead by example and embrace every moment of her young life. In retrospect, it's a little ironic that I set out on a course to lose weight and get healthy while my wife was gaining weight, albeit baby weight. Naturally, she was very supportive and the discussions about our respective weights provided some humorous moments throughout the pregnancy.

This was also the time that I became committed to dusting off the concept of JumpSnap, The Ropeless Jump Rope, that I had bouncing around in my head for about seven years since 1997. The concept of the product is to harness all the calorie-burning benefits of a traditional jump rope while removing the part that frustrates most of us, the rope. At that time, I didn't have the skill set, money or the motivation to pursue its development. This was probably a blessing in disguise. Now, I had a much deeper personal motivation to create and develop this new fitness product and figured what better way to test it than on myself. After many trips to Home Depot and Toys R Us to preview parts and materials, I had created a working prototype that was good enough that I could begin to test the benefits of JumpSnap. I figured I would use the product in its crude form while the designers did their job to make it more appealing for the mass market.

The Ah Ha's of Weight Loss

When I first started my JumpSnap workouts, I could barely do one minute without stopping and couldn't do more than five or six minutes combined. I immediately knew I was onto something by the pure sweat I was enjoying in just a few minutes of the exercise. It was also one of the first times in many years I had stuck with anything. I would JumpSnap right after I got home from work and before dinner, so I had no excuse. I literally would walk in the door, greet Susan, put on my shorts and sneakers and head down to the basement for five to ten minutes of JumpSnap while watching the evening news. I really think this is one of the key contributing factors that enabled me to stick with it because I was literally done before my brain could even rationalize why I couldn't work out that day. Compared to the standard heath club membership, I was done and showered in the same amount of time it would have taken me to drive to the gym, change clothes, and scout out an open machine. For me, like everyone else out there who struggles to exercise regularly, time was the number one stumbling block.

As the months went on and the formal development of JumpSnap came together, the weight kept coming off. When I started in the fall of 2004, I reached my heaviest weight of 205 pounds and I had a goal weight in mind of 175 pounds by my birthday of April 14, 2005. This gave me roughly six months to lose 30 pounds. I felt that was achievable, and the more weight I lost due to my JumpSnap workouts fueled my appetite to learn more about healthy living. Remember what I said previously about "knowing" and "understanding"? The progress I was gaining encouraged me to become a student of healthy living which ultimately make up the Ah Ha's in this book.

I was JumpSnapping five days a week feeling good about my exercise when I realized I needed to focus equally on my intake, specifically my calories. Since nutrition is half the equation for sustainable weight loss, I became a student of the basics. Creating my own calorie log was an eye-opening experience and allowed me to maximize my exercise with reduced calorie nutrition. By the time my self-imposed goal of April 14 arrived, I weighed 175 pounds, that was a full 30 pounds lighter than my previous weight, and people were noticing. I had to purchase an entirely new wardrobe that brought me back to my 34 inch waist pants. I was ecstatic.

I really had a lot of positive momentum going and realized my initial goal was just phase one. I wanted more. I was gaining a deeper knowledge of how it all worked together that made me more confident to laugh at the millions of myths that pop up in the market every day.

My next goal was to get back to my high school weight of 155 pounds, which candidly I wasn't sure I could do. (I only share that with you because bouts of self doubt are part of the process, so don't beat yourself up over every little imperfection.) After two periods of plateau, I was able to lose the remaining 20 pounds by the spring of 2006. All in all, it took me about a year and a half to lose the entire 50 pounds. That may not stack up to the statistics of the next bogus diet of the week, but this is real weight loss for real people.

Naturally, my personal story differs from yours. Perhaps you are a dedicated mother who always puts her family's needs first and literally forgets about her own health and wellness. Or maybe you are a busy father who struggles to juggle the demands of the office with those of raising a family. Or maybe you've been overweight your entire life and have grown to accept it as if it's genetic. Regardless of our stories, we are all in the same place. We want a change and are willing to work at it and take the common sense approach to healthy living. The basic principles of weight loss apply to us all. That's the good news. The better news is that you will be successful if you invest the necessary time, energy and discipline to incorporate these Ah Ha's into your daily life.

You and the Mirror

Remember, it took me seven years to amass the weight, so being able to take it off in under two years is a pretty good return, if you ask me. The best news of all is that I've been able to keep it off for over two years and know exactly which levers to pull if I'm not feeling as fit as I should. The weight loss is great, but the knowledge and confidence you will gain along the way is really what I want to share with you in this book.

With this goal in mind, to encourage you to maximize your progress, I've included a brief workbook component following each Ah Ha which I've titled "You and the Mirror." The name illustrates what this journey is all about. The intent of this workbook section is to inspire you to look closely at yourself (in the mirror) and take immediate action to apply each Ah Ha. I want you to enjoy the book, but more importantly, I want you to apply the contents to best suit your goals. I want you to be able to go back and reference a given Ah Ha when you need it. Write in the margins and take notes about key concepts to help you absorb the material. If you can use my experiences and adapt them to your life, then I have achieved my ultimate goal. I want you to advance beyond the head-nodding stage and take an active role in your own success. As the description implies, at the end of the day, it's you and the mirror that determine your level of success.

Before we jump in, let's take a deep breath and prepare ourselves to absorb the information. Don't overcomplicate it. You've probably heard some of the stuff before, but what I want you to focus on is the simplicity and how to incorporate it into your daily life. Let's have some fun and enjoy these Ah Ha moments together. Expect success, but don't expect it overnight. I look forward to hearing about your personal achievement and doing your part to help lead by example in the pursuit of healthy living.

About the Author

Brad LaTour is a....

	YES	NO
Trainer to the Stars	☐	☒
High Performance Athlete	☐	☒
Nutritionist	☐	☒
PhD in Exercise Science	☐	☒
Health Club Owner	☐	☒
Certified Personal Trainer	☐	☒
Fitness Model	☐	☒
Hard working guy in his late 30s, husband, father of two, first-time inventor, first-time author, and someone who gained seven to eight pounds per year over the course of about seven years who got fed up and decided to make some life changes in pursuit of a healthy lifestyle.	☒	☐

Now, 50 pounds lighter and 6 inches slimmer in his waist, Brad wants to share with you what he learned throughout his almost two-year journey towards a healthier lifestyle.

Ah Ha #1: Magic Pills Just Don't Exist

We need to keep it real. Even though it may be painful to accept, we need to be in the right frame of mind to properly absorb the upcoming Ah Ha's. To do that, we need to debunk the most destructive myth out there and be fully committed that we finally understand and accept it:

There is no magic pill.

Yes, that's right, there is no pill to swallow to make you lose weight. I'm sorry to destroy the myth, but it's true. Let me ask you, if all the magic pills, potions and lotions work, why then is obesity the #1 health crisis in America? Companies are making billions of dollars on these products because they are great at marketing them, but the products themselves obviously aren't working. Please stop wasting your hard-earned money on gimmicks and schemes.

If you're a serial purchaser of the next great weight loss miracle, STOP. Take a deep breath and ask yourself, "Am I committed to making a change?" If not, then don't spend your money on any product, JumpSnap included.

I admit that as I flip through the TV channels I do watch the infomercials featuring some of these weight loss miracles, primarily because I can't believe people actually pick up the phone and throw away their hard-earned money. Until you're honest with yourself and are committed to making the change, you're going to continue to fuel these inferior products. I know it's tempting to make impulse decisions with your heart while not listening to your head.

One of the reasons these magic pills attract attention is simply the sheer confusion in the marketplace. On one hand, you have clinicians, nutritionists and doctors, seemingly credible experts, talking at a higher level than most people can comprehend. They sound impressive as they bring plenty of science and studies to the discussion, but that doesn't mean it's any easier to understand. In fact, all those medical studies often just make us question where to start which usually ends up being no where.

On the other hand, you have the magic pill spokesperson telling you outright lies. You know the ones—promises of rock-hard abs or cellulite-free thighs or even cleaner intestines. The marketing is so perfect that you tell yourself, "Well, maybe it does work" or "They wouldn't be able to make those claims if it didn't do that." We are so tempted by the marketing of these products, it's no wonder that it's a multi-billion-dollar-per-year market. Promotions by the so-called scientific and medical experts and slick sales people make it a very confusing marketplace, especially since these "experts" are often paid endorsers who hope to lend credibility to the product. Naturally, we want to believe and buy into the easiest solution.

Often connected to one of these mysteriously effective magic pills is some sort of exotic diet making the same miracle weight loss claim. Sorry, these don't work either. Although you may have heard these fun facts about diets before, they are worth restating:

* **Fact: 95% of all diets fail**—That means that when you claim you're going on a diet, you're actually signing up to fail. I don't know about you, but I resist knowingly entering the failure business. However, that's exactly what you do when you go on a diet. We'd all like to believe that we'll be part of the 5% who succeed, but the odds

are severely against us. Try applying these types of "success" rates to anything you do in life, and then decide if you would proceed with the decision. For example, would you buy any household item or a car or toy if there was a 95% chance it was going to break? Would you buy any perishable item from the grocery store if it had a 95% chance of rotting or getting stale before you had a chance to eat it? Would you invest in a business if you knew it had a 95% chance of going bankrupt? Probably not.

* Fact: 75% of the people who lose weight on a diet actually gain more weight back than they initially lost. — UGH! If the 95% statistic didn't scare you off from starting a diet, this one certainly should. Think about that for a minute. You have a three out of four chance of gaining more weight on your next diet. Huh? Why in the world would anyone start a diet in the first place if they knew the odds are this bad?

I challenge you to fine tune your senses. When you hear some version of the next weight loss miracle in the form of a pill or something similar, listen to the disclaimer. Or better yet, take a stroll down the weight loss aisle of any drug store and read the fine print on the packages. Every single one of them says "with appropriate diet and exercise." Save your money on the illusive magic pills, because without the diet and exercise, they don't work. Go to the real solution, which is nutrition and exercise. I'm really sorry if I burst your magic pill bubble, but we needed to get this out of the way early so we can move on to the real work of sustainable weight loss. Ready, let's dig in.

You and the Mirror

1. Go to your local drug store and read the packages of the alleged weight loss pills. How many don't include some fine print about 'use in conjunction with diet and exercise'?

2. Watch an infomercial for a miracle weight loss product and write the disclaimer below:

3. Find an ad in a magazine for a weight loss pill and write the disclaimer below:

4. Sign the contract below:

I accept that there is no magic pill. I commit to achieving sustainable weight loss through exercise and nutrition.

_____ (signed) _____ (date)

Ah Ha #2: It's Simple Math—
Calories Consumed vs. Calories Burned

Now that you understand there is no magic weight loss pill, it's time to focus on the facts that *can* help you achieve your goal. Ah Ha #2 is actually so simple you may miss it. I did.

> Weight loss results from burning more calories per day than you consume.
> Or in mathematical terminology:
> Weight loss = calories burned > calories consumed

I have a bachelor's degree from the great Penn State University. I've traveled the country extensively and have been relatively successful in most aspects of my life. I've managed countless budgets, reviewed plenty of balance sheets, and built several pro-formas. I understand basic mathematical computations, especially as related to business. Even as a kid I knew that to make a profit, I had to take in more money than I spent (profit = income > expenses). Most of us use basic math to manage our household budget. We understand how much money comes in each month and pay the monthly bills accordingly based on our income. It is easy to understand the give and take relationship with numbers like those.

When it came to weight loss, it took me years to figure out such a simple mathematical equation (weight loss = calories burned >

calories consumed). Perhaps it took me so long to understand this concept because the consumer marketing industry had programmed me to believe it was much more complicated.

For years I thought I could eat whatever I wanted and not gain weight as long as I was active. I was focusing on calories burned without paying attention to calories consumed. A lucky few can eat as much of anything that they want and not gain weight, but to lose weight successfully or to maintain our current weight, the majority of us need to understand the mathematical relationship between how many calories or fuel we consume vs. the number of calories we burn.

During my first two months of using JumpSnap, I focused only on calories burned, not on calories consumed. Granted, this is 50% better than most folks. However, as I learned more about the nuts and bolts of weight loss, I realized that to maximize my workouts I needed to also understand the amount of fuel (number of calories) that was entering my body. I began to track my caloric intake by using a simple spreadsheet, which I affectionately dubbed my Calorie Truth Table.

Here's the Truth Table for a week in March of 2005. It shows the various metrics I was most interested in tracking along with the summary view of each day by category.

Ah Ha #2: It's Simple Math

	M	T	W	TH	FR	Weekly AVG	SAT	SUN
	3.14	3.15	3.16	3.17	3.18		3.19	3.20
Breakfast								
Calories	395	450	340	355	290	366	288	368
Fat Grams	2	13	13	4	13	9	17	18
Carbs	80	53	27	64	23	49.4	18	30
Fiber	5	6	6	9	3	5.8	12	9
Protein	10	23	21	11	19	16.8	15	16
Lunch								
Calories	500	840	580	795	580	659	960	660
Fat Grams	8	31	9	37	9	18.8	48	28
Carbs	0	84	84	62	84	62.8	84	76
Fiber	2	5.5	8	5	8	5.7	8	6
Protein	8	29	36	49	36	31.6	46	19
Dinner								
Calories	700	650	1108	352	1180	798	1238	348
Fat Grams	33	20	14	12	33	22.4	17	14
Carbs	46	80.5	73	10	124	66.7	74	25
Fiber	8	6.5	4	9	6	6.7	1	4
Protein	26	26.5	78	47	47	44.9	33	28
Snacks								
Calories	825	470	350	260	360	453	0	199
Fat Grams	46	17	13	7	15	19.6	0	7
Carbs	70	61	41	39	47	51.6	0	31
Fiber	10	6	3	3	5	5.4	0	4
Protein	37	23	20	14	13	21.4	0	5
Daily Total								
Calories	2420	2410	2378	1762	2410	2276	2486	1575
Fat Grams	89	81	49	60	70	69.8	82	67
Carbs	196	278.5	225	175	278	230.5	176	162
Fiber	25	24	21	26	22	23.6	21	23
Protein	81	101.5	155	121	115	114.7	94	68

As you can see, this basic spreadsheet only tracks five inputs—calories, fat grams, carbs, fiber and protein. These are the key criteria I think are the most important in managing weight. (More details on these metrics will be covered in Ah Ha #14.) I intentionally kept the chart simple so that I would stick with it. Over the years I've realized that if the worksheet is time consuming and too complex,

I won't use it for very long. I resisted the urge to track too much. I knew the importance of building a foundation with only a few items to track. Once I had these down, I knew I could always add more later as my desire to learn grew.

Let's see what we can learn from the Truth Table for this particular week. First, note the variance between days. Total calories consumed for Saturday exceeded Sunday's by almost 1,000 calories. Next, notice the calorie difference on some of my dinner meals. Again, I consumed almost double the number of calories for dinner on Wednesday than I did on Tuesday. Also, on Thursday for dinner I consumed far below my average at only 352 calories. That more than likely indicates my meal for that evening was one of those prepared diet meals. Looking a little deeper however, I gave all the calories saved for Thursday dinner back on Friday night which means I probably ate a pizza. Again, without the actual numbers in front of you, it's simply too easy to guess, and guessing will always lean in your favor.

Snacks are a big deal in the game of weight loss. Most of us intuitively think of snacks as unhealthy because we associate them with poor food choices (such as chips, candy, cookies, and processed crunchy things). On the contrary, selecting healthy snacks (such as fruit, raw vegetables, hummus, and nuts) and eating every two to three hours will have a dramatic impact on your weight loss. Healthy snacks are a key ingredient for controlling your appetite between meals while keeping the fire of your metabolism burning. ("Metabolism" is a collection of chemical reactions that take place in the body's cells to convert the fuel in the food we eat into the energy needed to power everything we do, from moving to thinking to growing.)

Ah Ha #2: It's Simple Math

Take a look at my snacks section for this week.

Snacks	M	T	W	Th	F	Avg	Sat	Sun
Calories	825	470	350	260	360	453	0	199
Fat Grams	46	17	13	7	15	19.6	0	7
Carbs	70	61	41	39	47	51.6	0	31
Fiber	10	6	3	3	5	5.4	0	4
Protein	37	23	20	14	13	21.4	0	5

As a reminder, I consolidated this section so it actually represents my morning and afternoon snacks for each day. Notice the difference in my Monday snack total of 825 calories and my Thursday snack total of only 260 calories. That's over a 3X difference, and it's the same week. I hope you're beginning to see the value of documenting your fuel intake.

Lastly, let's review just the weekend.

Daily Total	SAT	SUN
Calories	2486	1575
Fat Grams	82	67
Carbs	176	162
Fiber	21	23
Protein	94	68

Most people eat differently Monday–Friday than they do on the weekend because during the week they follow a routine. Notice the variance between the total calories consumed on Saturday versus Sunday. What do you see? Yes, it's obvious that I consumed a lot more calories on Saturday, most notably my dinner meal.

Rather than dwell on the negative, how about some high-5s for how I rebounded on Sunday with almost 1,000 fewer calories! This is a significant point because it demonstrates real life and what I call the "levers" to affect change. ("Levers" are items you can use to your advantage to achieve results or ways to change negative factors into positive ones.) I know I went a little over board on Saturday, but rather than curl up in a ball of defeat, I rebounded with a frozen prepared dinner on Sunday night. The game of weight loss will not be won in single meals or days or even weeks but rather in a lifetime of consistent choices. The sooner you understand and use the levers, the quicker you will enjoy success.

This type of analysis can be an eye opener. Do you think I would have known these variances had I not tracked the calories and written them down? Let me answer that one—not a chance! Now I think you understand why the name of this spreadsheet is the "Calorie Truth Table."

When you lay out your consumption like this, you've begun the commitment process. Trust me, you might unknowingly lie to yourself or, for some of you, blatantly lie to yourself because you're still scared of the truth. That's perfectly understandable, but the key is to value the power in seeing the numbers. Focusing on the numbers helps you remove some of the emotion of the food itself which can also be an empowering part of the equation. You'll also be able to review trends, obvious weaknesses, some potential strengths and, of course, areas of opportunity.

In addition to the weekly summary view shown previously, I used a similar simple spreadsheet layout to track each day. I broke my consumption into breakfast, morning snack, lunch, afternoon snack and dinner. From this daily view I was able to obtain the summary data. Tracking my consumption in these categories made me more aware of how often I was eating. In my research, industry experts almost unanimously agreed that we should eat five or six times per day or every 2.5–3 hours in an effort to keep our metabolism fired up.

Ah Ha #2: It's Simple Math

Nutritional Consumption Guide

Day	Friday
Date	3.18.05

Breakfast

Food Item	Calories	Fat Grams	Carbs	Fiber	Protein
Egg	90	5	1	0	8
Bacon (4 slices)	70	6	0	0	5
Potato roll	130	1.5	22	3	6
Sub Total	290	12.5	23	3	19

Lunch	Calories	Fat Grams	Carbs	Fiber	Protein
Quiznos turkey (12")	580	9	84	8	36
Sub Total	580	9	84	8	36

Dinner	Calories	Fat Grams	Carbs	Fiber	Protein
Digiorno pizza	960	33	111	6	45
Bud light (2)	220	0	13	0	2
Sub Total	1180	33	124	6	47

Snacks	Calories	Fat Grams	Carbs	Fiber	Protein
trail mix bar	140	4	25	2	3
Triscuits	120	4	20	3	3
Cheese	100	7	2	0	7
Sub Total	360	15	47	5	13

| **Daily Total** | 2410 | 69.5 | 278 | 22 | 115 |

By documenting my intake, I realized that much of what I was eating were wasted calories. They didn't always fill me up or leave me satisfied. They may have "tasted good," but they only left me wanting more because they didn't provide much nutritional value. We're going to explore this more in Ah Ha # 13 as it relates specifically to liquids. Using my simple layout allowed me to see if I was focusing on foods with higher protein and fiber content which made me feel less hungry and more satisfied. I also got into the habit of reviewing nutrition labels or at least stopping to consider what a food item truly contains. We're going to spend a lot more time on this topic in Ah Ha # 14 because understanding nutrition labels isn't always as easy as it sounds.

The good news about tracking food consumption is that it lays the foundation to learn more about what's in specific food items. Making that small step is significant towards the overall healthy living commitment. In fact, you're now beginning to understand how all these Ah Ha's work together. Taking the time to learn what I was consuming, and being honest with myself, enabled me to get the most out of my weight loss efforts. I was able to harness the calories burned through exercise to make a larger impact overall because I had reduced my calorie intake.

Understanding this concept of increasing the number of calories burned and decreasing the number of calories consumed is particularly helpful at every stage of the weight loss game, whether you are attempting to remove several years of added pounds like I was or trying to overcome the dreaded plateau to lose the final ten pounds. This approach is also particularly effective in maintaining a healthy weight level.

If you have never kept track of calories consumed or have not done it in a long time, I strongly encourage you to track your caloric intake for one month. Sure, it might be a pain, but what's one month in the grand scheme of things, especially if it leads you towards a healthier lifestyle. Keep it basic as I did, and don't worry about how good the chart looks because the content is the most important.

Several great Web sites can help you track your calories for free or for a small fee depending on your goals and depth of tools you're looking for. To assist you, here are some URLs you might be interested in viewing:

1. www.myfooddiary.com

Take the guesswork out of healthy living. By recording your food intake and your activity level, you will gain insight into the quality of the foods you are consuming, and you will have a better understanding of your metabolism and how food and exercise come into play. This Web site boasts a database of 50,000+ food items which can really make the task of calorie counting less painful. It also provides personalized reports based on your current health compared to future goals which I think can be motivating. It's only $9 per month with no contract and an easy cancellation process which I personally tested.

2. www.thecaloriecounter.com

This is a free site with no journal component to personalize your caloric intake or exercise. It's more of a Google-type layout whereby you enter the food group or item and it spits out the nutrition label. It's a no frills resource that allows you to count your calories.

3. www.caloriesperhour.com

This is another free site, but it is chockfull of information. There are several different calculators that help you determine how many calories you are burning as well as consuming. It's well organized and easy to use. This site is a good resource if you plan to maintain your calorie and exercise logs somewhere else.

4. www.nutritiondata.com

This is actually the site I used back in 2005 before it went through a major design makeover. It too is a free site that has the food items to help you calculate nutrition quantities, but it also makes suggestions. A special feature of this site is that it encourages you to explore food items that match your goals. To this day I still think about "fullness factor" which is a term it uses to help you select foods that make you feel fuller. Smart, right? Again, the only drawback is that you have to keep your journal separately from the site.

5. www.my-calorie-counter.com

This is an online diet and exercise journal that allows you to track your nutrient intake and find the calories you burn during exercise. It's actually free and seems to be very easy to navigate.

You and the Mirror

1. Write down the number of calories you think you consume on average each day. This will act as your mental baseline to compare your next seven days against.

   Breakfast: _____

   Morning Snack: _____

   Lunch: _____

   Afternoon Snack: _____

   Dinner: _____

   Total Calories: _____

2. Below, attempt to write down everything you ate yesterday including drinks, sauces, condiments, dressings—everything. This will prove to you that it's easy to forget or leave food items out, knowingly or not. BE HONEST!

   Breakfast:

   Lunch:

   Dinner:

Snacks:

3. Complete the daily Calorie Truth logs provided here for the next seven days starting with tomorrow's date as Day 1. Don't wait until you're finished with the book or next week or (insert favorite excuse here). Do it now and take action towards your own health. Remember, keep it simple and be honest. Trust me, this sounds much easier said than done, but it's the only way to accurately assess where you are today. Feel free to use some of the resources I outlined in this Ah Ha to further support your goals.

Ah Ha #2: It's Simple Math

Day _____   Date _____

Breakfast

Food Item	Calories	Fat Grams	Carbs	Fiber	Protein
Sub Total					

Lunch

	Calories	Fat Grams	Carbs	Fiber	Protein
Sub Total					

Dinner

	Calories	Fat Grams	Carbs	Fiber	Protein
Sub Total					

Snacks

	Calories	Fat Grams	Carbs	Fiber	Protein
Sub Total					
Daily Total					

The Ah Ha's of Weight Loss

Day _____   Date _____

Breakfast

Food Item	Calories	Fat Grams	Carbs	Fiber	Protein
Sub Total					

Lunch	Calories	Fat Grams	Carbs	Fiber	Protein
Sub Total					

Dinner	Calories	Fat Grams	Carbs	Fiber	Protein
Sub Total					

Snacks	Calories	Fat Grams	Carbs	Fiber	Protein
Sub Total					
Daily Total					

Ah Ha #2: It's Simple Math

Day _____ **Date** _____

Breakfast

Food Item	Calories	Fat Grams	Carbs	Fiber	Protein
Sub Total					

Lunch	Calories	Fat Grams	Carbs	Fiber	Protein
Sub Total					

Dinner	Calories	Fat Grams	Carbs	Fiber	Protein
Sub Total					

Snacks	Calories	Fat Grams	Carbs	Fiber	Protein
Sub Total					
Daily Total					

The Ah Ha's of Weight Loss

Day _____   Date _____

Breakfast

Food Item	Calories	Fat Grams	Carbs	Fiber	Protein
Sub Total					

Lunch	Calories	Fat Grams	Carbs	Fiber	Protein
Sub Total					

Dinner	Calories	Fat Grams	Carbs	Fiber	Protein
Sub Total					

Snacks	Calories	Fat Grams	Carbs	Fiber	Protein
Sub Total					
Daily Total					

Ah Ha #2: It's Simple Math

Day _____   Date _____

Breakfast

Food Item	Calories	Fat Grams	Carbs	Fiber	Protein
Sub Total					

Lunch

	Calories	Fat Grams	Carbs	Fiber	Protein
Sub Total					

Dinner

	Calories	Fat Grams	Carbs	Fiber	Protein
Sub Total					

Snacks

	Calories	Fat Grams	Carbs	Fiber	Protein
Sub Total					
Daily Total					

The Ah Ha's of Weight Loss

Day _____   Date _____

Breakfast

Food Item	Calories	Fat Grams	Carbs	Fiber	Protein
Sub Total					

Lunch	Calories	Fat Grams	Carbs	Fiber	Protein
Sub Total					

Dinner	Calories	Fat Grams	Carbs	Fiber	Protein
Sub Total					

Snacks	Calories	Fat Grams	Carbs	Fiber	Protein
Sub Total					
Daily Total					

Ah Ha #2: It's Simple Math

Day _____ Date _____

Breakfast

Food Item	Calories	Fat Grams	Carbs	Fiber	Protein
Sub Total					

Lunch

	Calories	Fat Grams	Carbs	Fiber	Protein
Sub Total					

Dinner

	Calories	Fat Grams	Carbs	Fiber	Protein
Sub Total					

Snacks

	Calories	Fat Grams	Carbs	Fiber	Protein
Sub Total					
Daily Total					

The Ah Ha's of Weight Loss

4. Now, use the data from your daily logs and complete the weekly summary "Calorie Truth Table" below:

	M	T	W	TH	FR	Weekly AVG	SAT	SUN
Breakfast								
Calories								
Fat Grams								
Carbs								
Fiber								
Protein								
Lunch								
Calories								
Fat Grams								
Carbs								
Fiber								
Protein								
Dinner								
Calories								
Fat Grams								
Carbs								
Fiber								
Protein								
Snacks								
Calories								
Fat Grams								
Carbs								
Fiber								
Protein								
Daily Total								
Calories								
Fat Grams								
Carbs								
Fiber								
Protein								

5. Review your 7-day logs and weekly summary log, and write below the "truths" they reveal:

   What are the trends?

   What are the weaknesses?

   What are some potential strengths?

   What are the areas of opportunity?

Ah Ha #3: How to Lose a Pound Mathematically

Congratulations on committing yourself to track your calories, fat grams, carbs, fiber, and protein for seven days. This big step lays the foundation for many upcoming Ah Ha's. Let's continue on to arguably the most important Ah Ha in the whole book.

As you begin counting calories and exercising regularly, it's helpful to understand the math behind your success. Drum roll, please, for Ah Ha #3:

In order to lose 1 pound, you must have a 3500 calorie deficit.

3,500 Calories

= 1 lb.

Now you know the missing link and the secret formula to weight loss that's been so elusive all these years. I think deep down we all want it to be more mysterious than a simple math equation. When it's this cut and dry, we can't say things like "I'm doing everything right and still not losing weight" or "I'm going to the gym five days per week and the scale isn't moving" or my personal favorite, "I'm only eating two meals per day and still gaining weight." Have any of you ever made these claims? I have.

Ah Ha #3: How to Lose a Pound Mathematically

If you want to lose weight and keep it off, you must understand the critical relationship between nutrition and exercise. Remember, weight loss is about the fuel (aka calories) and how much you consume versus how much you burn. If you're focused only on one or the other, you will most likely struggle as you attempt to build the tools for a sustainable weight loss and fitness program.

From my experiences, maximum results come when you truly understand the number of calories entering your body and the corresponding number you're burning. Truly understanding your caloric intake means counting everything that enters your mouth and not just the items you willingly list because you know they are good, healthy choices. If you don't understand this concept or are unwilling to be honest with yourself, the results will be flawed. I'm not saying you can't gain enough knowledge over time to make educated guesses about how many calories you're consuming without reading every single nutrition label, but most people need to build towards the ability to make a reliable educated guess as opposed to starting there. After all, you wouldn't think of trying to guess how much gas you have in your car. If you merely guess, you'd run the risk of overfilling the tank or running out of gas. Instead, you rely on gauges to indicate when you need to get gas. Same goes with nutrition—you need to track your intake and output so that you know when you are overfilling your "tank" or if you need to refuel.

Let's once again take the logical approach. If you merely begin to understand what you're eating by leveraging the nutrition labels, you will be surprised by how close you can get to attaining your goal for daily total calorie consumption. Remember to use the Web sites and other resources mentioned in the previous Ah Ha to assist you in tracking your calories and other nutritional data.

Here's my caution—the moment you begin to see success because of your regular exercise and healthy eating, you may become slightly neurotic about counting calories. Don't worry, once you begin to understand the general nutritional value of certain foods as well as realize most of us are creatures of habit, you'll tend to rotate the same meals on a regular basis. Thus your neuroticism about counting calories should subside.

The natural tendency is to want to shift the blame away from ourselves, especially on a topic as emotional as weight loss. I'm sure the skeptics out there are saying, "What about the magic pill?' or "It can't be this basic!" However, it truly is this simple, so let's take a closer look at what the math is telling us. For example, if you consume 2000 calories a day for seven straight days and burn 2500 calories per day, you'll lose 1 pound (500 calorie deficit/day x 7 days = 3500 calorie deficit or one pound lost). Now for those of you who allow yourself a "cheat day" every week and go way overboard on what you consume, the math won't work. To lose one pound in seven days, you must have a 500 calorie deficit every day of the week for all 7 days—including your cheat day! A 500 calorie deficit for only 5 days or even 6 days won't do it.

Achieving the 500 calorie deficit EVERY DAY for a week is hard because our lives are often different Monday–Friday than they are on Saturday and Sunday. Illustrating what it takes to lose one pound in simple math terms makes it real. This is a great first step towards understanding how you can realistically achieve your goals. Naturally, the easiest way to achieve your goal is to reduce your current caloric intake and increase your calorie burn so you're leveraging both sides of the equation.

Now that you know that 3,500 calories equals a pound, you should be better able to hone in on your approach to weight-loss and fitness. In addition, you should have a better framework for setting more realistic goals. Sometimes we have an event coming up or a change in season or a vacation or potential life-changing event that has us highly motivated to lose weight. In situations like these, far too many of us set ourselves up for failure saying things like, "I'm going to lose ten pounds in the next two weeks." Perhaps this is why 95% of all diets fail to produce lasting results. Although losing ten pounds in two weeks can be done, that's an awfully tall order and one likely to end in disappointment. Think about it, that would be a 3500 calorie deficit x 10 pounds = 35,000 calorie deficit / 14 days = 2500 additional calories burned each day above what's being consumed. Again, not impossible, but highly unlikely and certainly not sustainable.

Follow the mathematical approach, then, and build a game plan based on daily calories consumed and exercise. Once you have a game plan, then you can set goals as to the weight you want to achieve by a certain date.

For the record, anyone who is losing one pound per week on a sustainable basis deserves a huge pat on the back. Although it may not sound like much, consistently losing one pound per week is a major accomplishment. If weight loss is your goal, I recommend you set your goal to lose one pound per week and resist the temptation to set your goal higher. Even if you are so fortunate to follow your new plan with supreme discipline and you exceed your goal, treat it as a bonus rather than as a requirement. Far too many of us set weight loss goals that are unrealistic causing us to struggle out of the gate, get disappointed and ultimately quit, so let's not allow that to happen to you.

You and the Mirror

1. Tear this out (fridge poster) or go to www.jumpsnapnation.com and print it and place it on your fridge as a reminder of this simple math equation.

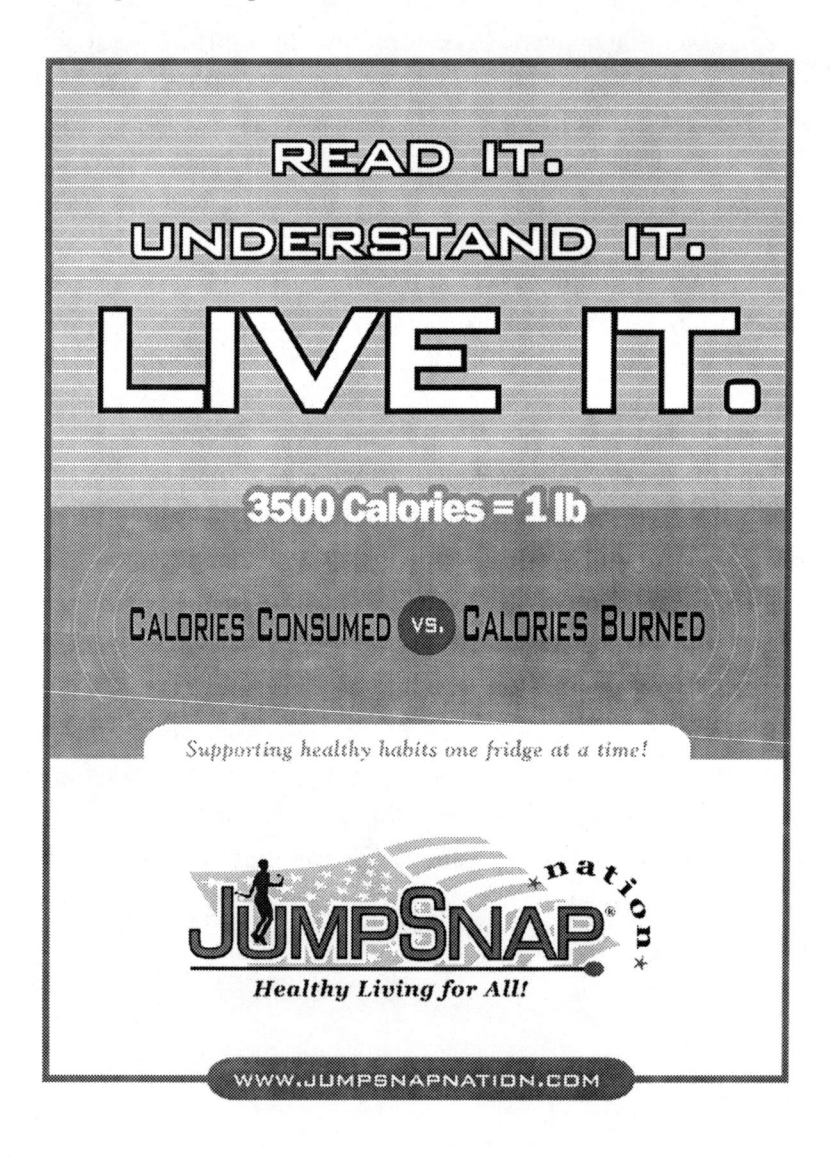

**READ IT.
UNDERSTAND IT.
LIVE IT.**

3500 Calories = 1 lb

CALORIES CONSUMED vs. CALORIES BURNED

Supporting healthy habits one fridge at a time!

JUMPSNAP® nation
Healthy Living for All!

WWW.JUMPSNAPNATION.COM

2. Randomly ask ten people one simple question, "How many calories equal one pound?" and document your findings. Don't accept "I don't know" but rather ask them to make a guess. You could also rephrase the question by saying, "If you wanted to lose one pound, how many calories would you have to burn?" Please email me your results to poll@jumpsnap.com so I can add your responses to those I have gathered.

_____   _____

_____   _____

_____   _____

_____   _____

_____   _____

Ah Ha #4: Exercise, Exercise, Exercise

Let's review the Ah Ha's so far:

1 — There are no magic pills.

2 — To lose weight, you need to burn more calories than you consume. (weight loss = calories burned > calories consumed)

3 — In order to lose one pound, you need a deficit of 3,500 calories. (3,500 calories = one pound)

Now with a firm grasp of these fundamentals, let's delve into the exercise side of the 50-50 exercise/nutrition equation.

As a society, we're falling woefully short when it comes to exercising regularly. One reason could be that we are enamored with progress and the latest, greatest technology. We want things to be "better, faster, stronger, and more efficient." We enjoy what the latest technology has to offer and are tempted to spend our spare time lying around and watching TV, sitting in front of a computer for hours or playing video games until the wee hours of the morning. Just because we can do these things doesn't mean that we should. Having access to these technologies doesn't give us a license to be lazy.

If it's not the technology, it's our busy schedules that become the reason. With long daily commutes to and from the office, it's

Ah Ha #4: Exercise, Exercise, Exercise

a struggle to make the time to exercise. What's more, when we're not working, we're spending time with family and friends pushing exercise further down the list of priorities. Granted, these are indeed legitimate life pressures we all face, but we must learn to overcome them.

However, progress and our busy schedules aren't the enemies that are sabotaging our weight loss and fitness efforts. We are. We all have 24 hours in a day. We can choose how we spend those hours, being active or being sedentary, or somewhere in between.

As you're starting to realize, I believe that to achieve a sustainable healthy lifestyle, you have to pay equal attention to exercise and nutrition. Combined, they are the keys to success.

How do you get started? Starting with nutrition and trying to lose weight by just changing your eating habits is challenging. Can it be done? Sure. Is it difficult? Absolutely. It's even harder to make it sustainable.

If you are having an honest discussion with yourself about making a change and want to lose an unwanted 10, 20, 50 or even 100 pounds, consistent exercise MUST be part of your strategy. As we've just agreed, there are no magic pills or plug-in gadgets to help you achieve **sustained** weight loss.

Therefore, you may have more success if you start with the exercise part of the exercise/nutrition equation. Exercise is actionable and more real. You feel the impact of exercise through sweat, fatigue, exhaustion, aches, and pains. If you work out, you feel good, you see results, your heart-rate is up, and you're sweating, thus you get immediate, tangible feedback. You'll start to see weight loss results. That's why I prefer to make regular exercise the pillar to long-term success.

I'm by no means saying that you'll achieve a sustainable healthy lifestyle through exercise alone. Focusing just on exercise and ignoring nutrition would be a flawed approach. Many people fall victim to that trap. They think they can consume whatever they want, just like they did perhaps when they were younger and more active. However, once their metabolism slows down, if they are only focusing on exercise and neglecting nutrition, they will most likely gain weight. I know from experience that working out intensively two weekends per month just doesn't get the results either. I think it's a much more natural progression to start with regular exercise and allow it to pique your interest in nutrition.

I also think it's easier for people to control exercise than it is to control nutrition. You can simply put on your running shoes and just start walking around the block regardless of your age or fitness level. Guess what? Your heart-rate will likely increase, and you might say something like, *"I don't know if I feel good or bad, but I feel different."* Contrast the walking example with a nutrition action. If you substitute eating broccoli for eating a pizza, you're just not going to notice much of a difference in how you feel. It would take many more nutrition actions (such as reducing calorie intake, eating more whole grain foods, and eating more fruits and vegetables, to name a few) before you would notice the results. The payoff from exercising tends to be much more tangible and immediate.

Set the expectation that you're going to have to work hard to get results. After all, if achieving fitness and weight loss results through exercising were that easy, everyone would be doing it successfully. Set the realistic expectation for yourself, work hard and be proud of your accomplishments. If you don't succeed in five days, keep at it realizing it takes some time. Remember, it took me about seven years to add on my additional weight, so to lose a big chunk of it in about six months is a great return on investment any way you slice it.

Ah Ha #4: Exercise, Exercise, Exercise

In fact, some of the best exercise opportunities are right in our own backyards. For example, if you live in a region that has hills or mountains, why not go hiking. Take a bicycle ride and explore your neighborhood or a local trail with your family or friends. Use the community pool and swim laps, or simply tread water which is a great workout. (Ever see the physique of a water polo player?) Conversely, if you live in an urban area, you can walk through a museum. Take a trip to the mall and park far away from your favorite store, thus forcing you to walk the extra distance—and no stopping at the food court! Hundreds of opportunities exist in our natural environment to support our exercise goals, and many of these activities cost little to no money.

I highlight this because many of us put too much pressure on ourselves by thinking that the only REAL exercise takes place at the gym. What a relief it is when we realize that exercising in our own surroundings can be just as effective. Think about it, truly incorporating exercise naturally into your daily routine can alleviate much of the unwarranted stress. It may even renew the enjoyment you used to experience when you exercised before you got wrapped up in the "you-have-to-belong-to-a-fitness-center" craze. Trust me, based on my experience, I know exactly how it feels when we pressure ourselves by narrowly defining exercise as activities that can only be performed in a traditional health club. Expand your definition of exercise by opening your eyes to your own environment, and change your behavior towards a lifetime of healthy living.

When I began my journey towards a healthy lifestyle, I started doing JumpSnap every day. I could only do about five to seven minutes in the beginning, but as my stamina improved, I increased my time. As my times increased, so did my pride in my accomplishments. I then added the hand weights into the handles which naturally helped build muscles in my back, shoulders, triceps and biceps. Then, from there, the results naturally motivated me to want more results.

To achieve more results, I introduced anaerobic exercises with the intent of building lean muscles. (Anaerobic exercises use muscles at high intensity and a high rate of work for a short period of time.) For example, I'm a big fan of push-ups in multiple forms: shoulder push-ups, regular push-ups, incline push-ups, decline push-ups, one arm push-ups, . . . you get the idea. Remember, push-ups cost no money, and you can do them anywhere. They will provide fantastic results which will boost your confidence. You'll never max out because you can always do more.

Other cost-effective exercises you can do are boot-camp style workouts. They typically incorporate tested exercises like walking lunges, squats, crunches, and a variety of core muscle-building activities. (The core muscles are the muscles in the body's center of gravity that support the spine and torso. These muscles initiate movement and are the main support of the body.) You can do them outside, inside, with a group, or by yourself. Again, you can do these anaerobic exercises to build lean muscle mass, and you don't necessarily need to go to a gym.

If you do have a fitness club membership, your choices are even more extensive. You can use a variety of machines for both aerobic and anaerobic exercises as well as free weights or dumbbells. Dumbbell work-outs are excellent because using dumbbells properly makes you focus on your form, provides resistance, and thus builds strength.

Exercising consistently will help you build the foundation for future success and improve your discipline. For me, results fueled my fire for more results. When I lost the first five pounds, I felt exhilarated. I immediately wanted to lose five more. I wanted to continue exercising because I knew it was working. It even drove my appetite for education. I wanted to learn more. This success-breeds-success component to weight loss often gets overlooked because we're so consumed with finding the one simple answer to solve our problems, and this one answer simply doesn't exist. Once you've been successful with one of your weight loss and fitness efforts, you need to keep searching for ways to continue achieving even more.

Exercise builds the foundation for sustainable healthy living. Allow exercise to jumpstart your desire for results. Doing so will help you develop a genuine interest to learn more about the power of combining exercise and nutrition. You'll then begin to see the proven benefits of applying the 50-50 exercise/nutrition equation.

You and the Mirror

1. List below the activities you do that you consider to be exercise:

2. Put a check mark beside the days you exercised in the last 7 days.

   Day 1 _____

   Day 2 _____

   Day 3 _____

   Day 4 _____

   Day 5 _____

   Day 6 _____

   Day 7 _____

3. How many times did you exercise in the last 30 days.

4. In addition to going to the gym, running or the more standard exercises, list ways you can incorporate exercise into your daily routine:

5. List below times you exercised with family or friends and what you did:

Ah Ha #5: Make Fitness a Budget Item

The best things in life aren't always free. As the saying goes, "You get what you pay for." Achieving your fitness goals requires not only a personal commitment but a financial commitment as well. When it comes to investing in a healthy lifestyle, don't shortchange yourself. Make fitness a budget item. Commit to spending a certain amount of money each month on fitness and exercise.

One way to stay motivated is to have some "skin in the game." The mere fact that you've put some money towards your fitness and exercise goals may provide additional incentive to stay with them. If you never spend money on fitness-related products, then you may find it far too easy to pack it in at the slightest excuse for not exercising. On days when you need that extra push to work out, and believe me, there will be those days, realizing you had already spent your hard-earned money on the tools to help you achieve a healthy lifestyle could be just the nudge you need. If you haven't invested any money in a membership, home workout program, personal training session or fitness workshop, you may find that it's just easier to rationalize your excuse. The realization that "I'm wasting money when I'm not exercising" can be a helpful reminder to get your good habits back on track. If you invest in yourself financially, you are more likely to invest in yourself mentally and physically further supporting the need to exercise consistently.

Ah Ha #5: Make Fitness a Budget Item

If financially feasible, you might consider joining a health and fitness club. They are a great resource because they provide you with different types of equipment all in one location for a monthly fee. For some people, one of the keys to sticking with a fitness program is variety. They get bored with the same old routine and eventually quit. A health club can make it easier to change workouts and increase intensity to help achieve greater results.

Fitness clubs also provide access to personal trainers. These trainers can help assess your fitness needs and set up a personalized training regimen that is balanced and may help you get more out of your workouts. Doing just one personal training session can help you cut through the clutter of which machines to use, when to use them, and in what sequence as well as how much weight or resistance is appropriate. The trainer can also demonstrate the proper form to cut down on possible injuries and provide maximum benefit to each exercise. From there you can gain the confidence you need to either continue with the trainer or go it alone without feeling lost or intimidated. Even if you can't afford to stick with a trainer on a regular basis, it's worth the money to do at least one session. To get maximum benefit from your session, prepare for your appointment by clearly articulating your fitness goals. Remember, it's your time and money, so don't be afraid to ask lots of questions and take notes.

In addition to the equipment and personal trainers, many clubs offer a wide range of organized classes, commonly referred to as Group Exercise. These classes typically offer a range of options from cardio to strength training while appealing to all fitness levels. The social aspect to fitness classes or even having a workout buddy may motivate you to stick with a fitness program. Some people go to the club to see other people and, therefore, have a greater incentive to show up because their "fitness friends" expect them to be there. Group exercise is also a more cost-effective option than one-on-

one personal training and often times is included in your monthly membership fee.

Health club memberships vary in price from $20 per month to $200 per month depending on the range of services they offer. Many of the nationally recognized brands offer a variety of payment plans to match your budget and goals. Since this is a highly competitive market, many clubs offer a free trial or charge a nominal fee to try the club out for one or two visits. Even if they don't formally offer something like this, ask them to let you work out for free or offer to pay $10 per visit for up to three visits so you can effectively evaluate the club.

Put it on your "to-do" list to visit one or more fitness clubs in your area to evaluate their ability to fit your needs. Then decide if joining the club would be beneficial and thus worth the financial commitment required. If you're uncertain about joining, the last thing you want to do is sign a membership contract and then have to deal with canceling it.

I caution you, however, not to use the "I'm-not-a-health-club-type-of-person" as an excuse. I say this as someone who has started and stopped four club memberships in my lifetime. At a minimum, joining a club can give you that short-term burst of motivation to get you back on track towards a healthy lifestyle.

If you've given the club option a realistic shot and it's still not motivating you, then simply think of other ways you can commit a specific dollar amount every month to spend on fitness. If you historically spent $30 per month on your health club membership and stopped going for whatever reason, take that same $30 and spend it on fitness products for your home. You may want to build a library of workout DVDs so that you can change up your workouts and keep them fresh. Or for variety, you may want to invest in a stability ball, resistance bands and perhaps some handheld dumbbells to work on muscle tone.

Ah Ha #5: Make Fitness a Budget Item

If you're not a DVD person, why not create your own workout you can do in the comfort and privacy of your own home. You can even design a routine you can do while watching your favorite TV show. You don't even need a lot of space to workout. Remember, keep it simple. If your workout is too complicated, you're likely not to stick with it. There are plenty of workouts you can do that provide excellent results by taking advantage of your own body weight so you don't need to invest in expensive machinery. Simple push-ups, leg lifts, jumping jacks, and other basic exercises have stood the test of time and can certainly do the trick.

Another option for investing in your health and wellness is to take a fitness vacation. I'm not talking about waking up a 5 a.m. to have a drill sergeant yell at you all day, but rather a vacation that involves physical activity. In the winter, consider going skiing or snowboarding. Taking a week each winter to enjoy the ski slopes is one of my favorite vacations. Regardless of the size of the mountain and level of difficulty, the mere elevation change will make your system work harder than normal. Remember—you'll enjoy this type of vacation much more if you're in shape prior to taking your first run down the mountain. This is more motivation to properly prepare a few months in advance of your trip.

If you prefer a warmer climate, how about a trip to a surf camp? That's right, surf camp. My good friends, Mike and Cindy Myers, went on a surf camp vacation to a place called Witch's Rock in Costa Rica. They liked it so much they've gone back four more times. I'm not certain Mike was necessarily focused on the physical aspect of the vacation, but he did confess that his abs, back and arms got a killer workout. As an encore this year, they spent 10 days kayaking in the Galapagos Islands. I think it's safe to assume they select vacation destinations that reflect their active and healthy lifestyle.

If you prefer a more traditional sightseeing vacation, pack your walking shoes. Do some research before you leave, and select a tour that incorporates plenty of walking. Think about it—you'll not only add exercise to your vacation, you'll feel less guilty as you indulge in the local cuisine. In fact, my parents have been teaching abroad for six weeks each summer for the past several years in places like England, Spain, Italy and Australia. They always include side trips on the weekends which entail lots of walking. After each trip, my dad would tell us how many miles they walked each day from one historical point of interest to the next. (It's funny, each time he told the story the distances seemed to get longer and longer.) I thought he was exaggerating, so we bought him a pedometer for Christmas. Now, I get a blow-by-blow description of each excursion with a detailed reference of the distance they walked to and from the sights. They have found that walking is an effortless way for them to get around the smaller villages, costs less, and allows them to stay fit while traveling. From a health perspective, they are getting daily exercise without having to think about it, which is always the most sustainable option.

You don't need to travel to exotic destinations or be away for days to reap the benefit of a fitness vacation. There are plenty of places that are closer to home that would accomplish the same goal. You simply need to go somewhere for a change of pace to be physically active that being at home doesn't provide or your daily schedule doesn't allow. What type of investment are your willing to make in your fitness budget—and your health? No matter how big or small, set a budget for wellness, stick to it, and most of all, remember, you're worth it!

You and the Mirror

1. Do you currently have a fitness budget and if so, how much do you spend per month?

2. If you don't have a fitness budget, what's a realistic amount to spend each month on fitness?

3. How much money do you currently spend on soda, coffee drinks and unhealthy treats each month?

4. List 5 fitness items you would like to purchase with your new fitness budget along with their approximate cost? (hint: It could be workout clothes, equipment, gym membership, new sneakers, sport watch, DVDs, registration for a 10k race, among others)

Item	Cost
a. _____	_____
b. _____	_____
c. _____	_____
d. _____	_____
e. _____	_____

TOTAL _____

5. What is the last item you purchased to help promote your fitness goals?

Ah Ha #6: Your Most Powerful Exercise Equipment—Your Brain

Forget the bench press, elliptical trainer, tread mill or even JumpSnap. When it comes right down to it, your most important piece of exercise equipment is your brain. The constant battle that rages between your ears can often determine success and failure along your journey toward achieving a sustainable, healthy lifestyle.

"Should I exercise this morning, or go back to bed?" "What about eating just one piece of that double chocolate chip birthday cake?" "I think I'll just workout for 20 minutes today instead of doing the 45 minutes I had planned. I can always make up for it tomorrow." "Why not super size my fast food meal—after all, it doesn't cost that much more?" Your brain can provide you the much needed discipline to exercise consistently and eat healthfully, or it can be the ultimate rationalizer giving you a free pass to give in and derail your best laid plans for achieving a healthy lifestyle.

Your success in achieving your goals hinges upon your ability to make the right decisions, your being disciplined to not stray off your path, your being accountable for your own success (and failure), and your steadfast commitment to make it happen. No piece of equipment can do these things for you. Your brain ultimately determines whether you succeed or whether you fail.

Ah Ha #6: Your Most Powerful Exercise Equipment—Your Brain

Let's say you want to achieve a certain number on the scale. If you don't see immediate results, the likelihood is that you're going to become discouraged, which can easily cause that number to go up rather than down. It's a process. It takes time. If you approach it the right way and stay committed with your workouts while understanding what you're consuming, it's you that's making that happen. Take credit for the progress that you initiate. It's not just about the miles on the treadmill or steps on the elliptical (or any other piece of equipment). It's you who is doing the reps and logging the time to achieve the results.

It's funny, but a lot of people ask me, "How does the JumpSnap actually know if you're really jumping?" I get that more often than you would think. My canned response is: "You can turn on the treadmill and walk away, but you don't get the same results as if you're actually running on it." My point is—you still have to do the work. You have to be committed to putting forth the effort. In addition, when you do the work, recognize that it's you that did it. Gaining that confidence builds the results, and those results lead to even greater results. At the end of the day, results are the one thing that will encourage you to keep exercising.

Two of my life moments will illustrate how my brain drove me to the point of *enough is enough* and thus was an integral part of my transformation. One occasion was the day I realized that my 36" pants were too tight to button, but I absolutely refused to buy pants with a 38" waist. "No way," my brain told me. "You have to do something about this!" It had been traumatic enough going from a size 34" to 36". At that point, I'd given myself a free pass to ignore my expanding waistline, but to go from a 36" to a 38" wasn't an acceptable option. At that moment I reignited my commitment to begin my weight loss and fitness regimen.

The other occasion happened a few months later when my wife and I found out we were pregnant with our first child. My brain at that point said, "How is it going to look if you try to raise healthy kids while you yourself aren't in good health?" I decided that I wanted to have an active fatherhood with my kids. I wanted to be able to run around, roll around, wrestle and do all the things you're supposed to do as a parent. Additionally, I wanted to lead by example which is my approach to everything in life. I live by the adage, "Don't just do what I say, but do as I do." These are two defining moments that have encouraged me down the path toward a sustainable, healthy lifestyle.

Your brain is powerful. If you think it, you can do it. Conversely, if you think you can't do it, you probably won't even try. When you allow your brain to support your success rather than to sabotage it, nothing can outweigh its influence.

Ah Ha #6: Your Most Powerful Exercise Equipment—Your Brain

You and the Mirror

1. List below the reasons you CAN'T be completely successful in leading a healthy lifestyle:

2. Now list the reasons you CAN be completely successful in leading a healthy lifestyle.

3. Now, go back and cross out all the reasons you can't, and then put a big star by the reasons you can.

4. How many times in the past two weeks did you intend to exercise? _____

5. How many times did you actually do it? _____

6. List below words that describe how you feel after you exercise:

   _____   _____
   _____   _____
   _____   _____
   _____   _____
   _____   _____

7. List below words that describe how you feel if you skip exercising:

   _____   _____

   _____   _____

   _____   _____

   _____   _____

   _____   _____

8. Describe below a time you had a great workout even though you had been tempted to postpone it for one reason or another (too tired, have to work, want to watch a TV show). Use this example as future motivation the next time you are tempted to blow off exercise:

Ah Ha #7: Muscle Is Your Friend

OK, you've seen my photo. So it's no surprise that with my intimidating 5' 8" 155 lb. frame, I probably won't be featured on the cover of *Men's Health* anytime soon. The end game for my fitness and weight loss efforts is not to be included in *People Magazine's* list of 100 most beautiful people. My guess is that the same holds true for you. My desire to build muscle specifically relates to my wanting to reap the benefits that having toned, strong muscles can provide.

When it comes to building muscle, you probably envision having washboard abs or bulging biceps. This would be an unrealistic expectation for most of us and would intimidate us into thinking, "Why even try!" For some reason we tend to think that there are only two options—we can either be ripped or flabby. You'll be relieved to know that regardless of your physique or level of fitness, you can benefit from strength training exercises that build muscle.

The overwhelming benefit of having strong muscles is that you can burn more calories more efficiently and you will feel better. In fact, for each pound of muscle in your body, you will burn an extra 50 calories per day. In a society that wants instant gratification, this is as close as you'll come to being able to burn calories while you sleep.

Another benefit is that having toned muscles will likely protect you against injury. Strength training and weight bearing exercises help slow down bone loss due to aging. In fact, exercising your bones makes them work harder, which helps them to build up bone mass. Greater muscle strength equates to stronger bones, so you may be less prone to fractures. Greater mobility and flexibility due to stronger muscles allows you to feel a greater connection to your body.

As mentioned elsewhere, seeing results makes you believe in the results—and inspires you to achieve even more. As you see and feel the muscles develop, you'll naturally appreciate what they can do for you. You'll feel more confident and have stronger self-esteem. The true payoff will be the positive impact on your long-term health.

I firmly believe in building good habits that are sustainable for a healthy lifestyle. For some of you, achieving a healthy lifestyle may mean that you need to slightly tweak some of your habits. For others who may have been battling obesity all of your life, you may need to make life-altering changes. Successfully building toned muscles can inspire you to go farther down the path of educating yourself on other health- and fitness-related tips.

Some of you may be saying, "But I don't have enough money to spend on light weight training." You don't need to spend tons of money on expensive weight bench systems or shell out money every month to the health club if you're on a tight budget. I guarantee that no matter how big or small you are, you only need a couple of ten pound dumbbells and your own body weight to accomplish your goals. If you can't afford the dumbbells, simply do the variety of push-ups we talked about previously in Ah Ha # 4. Trust me, you don't need to bulk up, but by all means, tone up! The benefits will be well worth the effort.

You and the Mirror

1. List some of the anaerobic or strength training exercises you've done in the past month.

   _____

   _____

   _____

2. If your list above is bare, list 3 exercises you can commit to for the next week to help build toned muscles:

   _____

   _____

   _____

3. What benefits do you think you'll enjoy with stronger, leaner muscles?

Ah Ha #8: Take the Stairs

"Take the stairs" is simply a metaphor for blending exercise into your daily routine. I could have named this Ah Ha, "Park farther from the store," or "Ride your bike to the park instead of driving your car." The principle is the same, no matter how I say it.

Start wrapping your mind around ways you can add exercise to what you do every day. A good place to begin is by taking the stairs instead of taking the escalator or elevator. I know, some of you have already made excuses about why taking the stairs just isn't realistic. "I work on the top floor of a high rise building. I can't climb 12 flights of stairs," or "I'd be too sweaty by the time I get to work." I won't debate you on the issue. I simply ask that you think about why you can do it, rather than why you can't. Take a deep breath and say, "If I had to, what could I do to add exercise to my daily routine?"

Sticking with the example of how someone who works on the 12th floor can incorporate exercise into their daily routine, let's take our collective breath and figure out some easy solutions. Let's consider ways to set ourselves up for success. Nobody wants to walk into the office sweating at 9:00 a.m. I know I certainly wouldn't want to. Here are some practical alternatives to consider:

A) When you arrive at work in the morning, park your car on the parking level farthest away from the entrance to the building. Then instead of taking the elevator in the parking

Ah Ha #8: Take the Stairs

garage, take the stairs from the garage to get to the lobby and then pick up the elevator from there.

B) When you're leaving work, get off the elevator in the lobby and take the stairs down to the parking garage and your car.

C) Once per week at the end of the day take the stairs down the full 12 flights.

D) Get off the elevator at the 10th floor one or two days per week when you come back from lunch and walk the remaining 2 flights.

E) Walk up three flights of stairs and then take the elevator the rest of the way.

OK, OK. You get the point. I could go on forever making simple suggestions about a fictitious office location on the 12th floor. The real importance of this exercise is not necessarily which one you pick but how you approach the activities in your daily life differently.

If you are at an airport, train station, or meeting with a crowd of people, do you follow the herd to the escalator or take the stairs? No seriously, answer the question. If you're anything like I used to be, you are programmed to position yourself to line up for the escalator. Depending on the event, being in a pack like this can feel like participating in a full contact sport. People are jockeying for position and with sharpened elbows are establishing their stake in the queue. Next time you're in a situation like this, take the stairs. Not only will you get more exercise, you'll probably have them all to yourself since 80% or more people will take the escalator.

"But what if I have luggage or an overstuffed briefcase? I can't possibly take the stairs then," you quibble. Even better, lug that suitcase up or down the stairs, and you'll add a new dimension of free weights to your real life exercise. The truth is that we all tend to be lazy, and we either don't know it or we won't admit it. Take a simple look around to observe how you maneuver your daily routine. I think you'll find a surprising number of opportunities to effortlessly blend daily life and exercise.

Now when I find myself in the "herd-of-people-lining-up-for-the-escalator" situation, I always take the stairs and mentally pat myself on the back. Yes, at times I want to take the escalator because I'm tired or I have some other excuse. The fact is, it's almost always faster to walk, and I instantly feel good about myself. I know this is such a small little example on your daily schedule, but when you can blend several of these individual examples into a lifestyle and philosophy, then you are on the right path towards sustaining a healthy lifestyle.

Let's try another one. Consider the people who circle a crowded parking lot for a spot closest to the door. In most cases it takes twice as long to select a spot than it would if they just parked farther away. It's amazing what people will go through to try to save a few extra steps. (I especially chuckle when people do this in the parking lot at their health club.) This is a great scenario because we all do it. I know, I can hear the excuses on this one, too. "I'm buying a lot of groceries, so I need to be close to the door," or "It might rain," or "I have parking karma." Take your pick for whichever excuse best suits you, or take them all if you're still shaking your head "yes." Consider these really crazy suggestions:

A) Park next to the cart corral area in the lot. It will actually be easier to unload your groceries or packages and then return the cart. These cart return areas are usually located an aisle or two away from the front door. Not only will it be easier to load your vehicle after you've finished shopping, but as a bonus you'll have gained a few extra steps—and burned a few more calories.

Ah Ha #8: Take the Stairs

B) Unless you're the wicked witch from the Wizard of Oz, you don't need to worry about a little rain. Just take that great invention called an umbrella or even a rain coat with you. Please don't get in the habit of blaming the weather for your lack of exercise. It starts with your not wanting to run errands because of the weather and can easily grow into not exercising outside because it's too hot, too cold, too wet, too windy, too humid, or any other unfavorable atmospheric condition.

C) So you say that your excuse for circling the lot is that you have parking karma—you know that if you drive around long enough a prime spot will open up just as you get there. You can then snap it up before someone else beats you to it. My wife says I have parking karma. I can usually find a parking spot without any problem. Perhaps that's because I'm never looking for a front row spot! I choose to park farther away so that I can squeeze in just a bit more exercise as I walk a few more steps to get from my car to the store. Stop wasting your karma on finding a parking spot—save it for your workouts!

Consider other every day opportunities to help add to your daily calorie burn. How about lifting items to help build lean muscle mass? Whether it's groceries or your kids, literally hundreds of items around us could easily complement reps of dumbbells at the gym.

I once shared a fun example of how to work exercise into everyday life on my blog. As you may know, I live in Annapolis, MD not far from downtown. The City Dock area of downtown is a beautiful setting on the Severn River and Chesapeake Bay with shops and restaurants lining the brick street appropriately named, Main Street.

One of my favorite morning activities is to take my daughters to the City Dock to get coffee for me and other treats for them. It's a great start to the day and yields some quality bonding time with the girls while Mom gets a well-deserved break. When my oldest daughter Cate was about 18 months old, she didn't want to get into the stroller right away. Rather than completely fight her on it, we usually made a deal that I would push her down to the City Dock and then she could get out and walk around, feed the ducks, and then walk home. I knew while I was negotiating this deal that she wouldn't be able to walk the whole way home. I'd have to carry her part of the way. How much running around we did at the City Dock would usually determine how far she could make it before she'd voice the proverbial "up please."

Our kids are the most loveable free weights available. Carrying them is an excellent way to build up your upper body. I'm serious, when you're carrying your kids you're actually carrying around an extra 20, 30 or even 40 pounds on your shoulders. Just like any weight lifting exercise, be conscious of your form so you don't injure yourself while gaining maximum benefit from the kid-lifting.

These few examples illustrate my point—it's amazingly easy to insert some form of exercise into your daily routine. Don't unduly pressure yourself to make it to the gym if your schedule is already over booked.

I'm not asking you to leave your car at home and take your bike to work, although that would be an incredible opportunity if it were feasible. All I'm asking is that you start with some small victories like taking the stairs and parking farther away from the front door and build in other exercise opportunities from there.

Making these changes will consciously cause you to think about having even better alternatives. That way, when something comes up and you can't make it to the gym, you won't get behind on your workout schedule because you've trained yourself to incorporate daily exercise into everyday life. When you get to that point, we're talking about some major Ah Ha's that will last a lifetime.

Ah Ha #8: Take the Stairs

You and the Mirror

1. List some of the ways you've blended exercise in with your everyday activities during the past seven days.

   1. _____
   2. _____
   3. _____
   4. _____
   5. _____
   6. _____
   7. _____
   8. _____

2. List some of the ways you can add even more exercise to your everyday activities during the next seven days.

   1. _____
   2. _____
   3. _____
   4. _____
   5. _____
   6. _____
   7. _____
   8. _____

Ah Ha #9: Fast Food Isn't New — The Lack of Exercise Is.

"It's the restaurants' fault." Are you kidding me? Nothing irritates me more about our society than the frivolous law suits that claim it's McDonald's or another fast food establishment's fault we're getting fat. C'mon, let's be accountable for our actions. If we're searching for whom to blame for our obesity epidemic, let's begin by looking in the mirror. Fast food has been around a long time. The first McDonald's was opened over 50 years ago. Fast food is simply not the problem. Whether it's our sedentary lifestyle or overflowing schedules leaving us too tired to exercise, we're just not as active as we should be.

When I was a kid, it was a treat to go to McDonald's after a game. We didn't go every week, and we certainly didn't let it replace a sensible dinner at home. Granted the portions served today may be larger than they were when I was growing up, but fast food restaurants and the temptation to eat fast food has existed for over half a century.

Simply stated, as a society, obesity is becoming so prevalent because we aren't getting enough exercise. We've deemphasized the importance of school gym classes. We've cut after school programs for budget reasons. We've allowed our kids to choose TV and electronics over backyard pick-up games. It's no wonder that our children do not recognize the importance of some consistent physical activity. After all, that's the message we're sending them, intentionally or not. With that type of upbringing, how can we expect them to all of sudden make regular exercise an integral part of their adult life?

To further support my point, a recent study published in the *Journal of American Medical Association* and funded by The National Institute of Child Health and Human Development shocked even me. It's apparently one of the largest studies of its kind tracking about 1,000 kids at various ages from 2000 to 2006.

The report states that while 90% of 9-year-olds are getting at least two hours of exercise most days, that number plummets to a mere 3% for kids that are age 15. Think about that for a minute. In just six years, children went from running around on the playground to lifeless on the couch.

Even more alarming, the study suggests that two out of three teenagers don't get the government's recommendation of the daily minimum of one hour of moderate to vigorous exercise. This is based on activity during the week, but surely it would be better on the weekends, right? Wrong! In fact, the activity level of teenagers got worse. Only about 17% of the 15-year-olds were active for an hour on Saturday and Sunday. Again, that's less than one out of five kids who are embracing their weekends and making the most of their free time by playing a pick-up game or riding a bike or going swimming.

I don't know about you, but when it comes to what the government recommends, I view that as the absolute lowest of the low, and we're even falling woefully short of that. Although not included in the study, I think it would be easy to argue that teenagers, especially the early teens, are precisely the age group that need the exercise the most since they are going through so many other difficult challenges associated with puberty. Exercise is the one proven stress reducer that allows these kids to better handle a notoriously awkward time of development, yet regular exercise is not happening.

We must continue to encourage an active lifestyle, for ourselves and for our children. Exercise opportunities come in so many shapes and sizes. In addition to the traditional health club, we can participate in countless organized sports or hike or dance or walk or anything we can think of that gets our heart rate up. I realize not everyone has the desire to be the star player on a sports team, but you have many other options to choose from. So, everyone get up, get out, and get moving! That's the way to fight obesity in your household.

You don't need to totally avoid fast food. Just recognize it for what it is and what it is not. It is not the ideal choice for a low calorie, nutritious meal option. If you're going to indulge in fast food, order sensibly. Understand what the menu has to offer you, or perhaps do some research before you go. Use their corporate Web site to review nutritional values so that you can make smart choices.

Because obesity has become an epidemic, almost every major fast food chain offers some healthier options. For example, some menus include salads or a grilled chicken sandwich instead of a deep fried one. Quiznos and Subway offer some low fat, low calorie sandwich choices.

Be careful—just because it's marketed as a healthy option doesn't always mean it is. Salads are usually a great option, but they don't give you a free pass. Read the nutritional information before you chomp. Some of these allegedly healthy salads have more calories and fat grams than their evil deep-fried and grilled siblings.

Also, recognize that some of your "forgotten" calories (calories that you forget to count) come in the form of liquids, dressings, condiments, and other items that are loaded with calories. From my own experience, we can easily eliminate these wasted calories from our consumption. Try this the next time you find yourself pulling up to the drive-thru window at a fast food restaurant. Instead of ordering the super-jumbo-gigantic-value-meal, order the sensible meal—the salads, chicken sandwiches, a side order of fruit instead of fries, or whatever nutritional option they have to offer. Ask them to leave off the mayonnaise, dressing, butter, bacon bits, or any other calorie-laden extras. Don't be embarrassed to get a kid's small hamburger or kid's portion of chicken nuggets. (Actually, the kid's meals today are the same size as the regular burger and fries were when I was growing up.)

For those of you for whom time is your biggest challenge, plan your food choices ahead of time. Think about what you'll be doing for the next half a day. If you're going to be in the car, take with you a handful of nuts, some sort of granola or cereal bar, an apple, a banana, or almost any piece of fruit that can travel with you. You'll have something nutritious available to eat. That way you won't feel so stressed out, and you'll be less likely to eat impulsively. The fuel you put in your body helps you in many aspects of your life. It's well worth it to invest a couple of minutes each day as you're arranging your schedule to determine when and where you are going to eat.

Additionally, try eating nutritional snacks multiple times throughout the day. You'll avoid building up a huge hunger pang that you'll have to satisfy. If you wait until you're really hungry before you eat, you're likely to choose something you think you want, rather than selecting the more nutritious option.

Making exercise an integral part of your daily life, choosing nutritional food options, planning ahead for what you're going to eat, and keeping hunger under control by eating the right type of foods frequently are all common sense, logical approaches to achieving a sustainable healthy lifestyle.

You and the Mirror

1. List below what you are doing to make exercise an integral part of your daily life:

   _____

   _____

   _____

   _____

2. Fast Food Log—Complete the following information about your most recent fast food experience:

   Name of the fast food restaurant: _____

   Date: _____

   Time of day _____

   Items eaten (Remember to include the condiments and extras)

   _____

   _____

   _____

   _____

3. Based on your answer to question #2, guess how many calories were in the food you ate:

   Guess: _____ calories consumed

Ah Ha #9: Fast Food Isn't New — The Lack of Exercise Is

Now go to the corporate Web site to determine how many calories you actually consumed.

Actual: _____ calories consumed

How does your guess compare to your actual?

What insight did you gain?

4. Using the same restaurant or one of your most frequent fast food stops, list below an alternative menu choice they offer with reduced calories and lower fat. (Most major chains list their nutritional value on their Web site.)

Reduced calorie, lower fat menu items you could choose:

Item	Calories	Fat grams
_____	_____	_____
_____	_____	_____
_____	_____	_____
_____	_____	_____

Ah Ha #10: Focus on Nutrition, Not on Diet

Take a deep breath, and let it out. For those of you who didn't think I was serious, let's do it again. Ready—big deep breath in, fill those lungs, and let it out. Excellent! We've spent the past few Ah Ha's focusing primarily on exercise. Now let's switch gears and chat about the other critical side of the equation–nutrition.

Let's begin by reprogramming ourselves on the choice of words we use. I want you to delete the word "diet" from your vocabulary. Replace it with the word "nutrition" instead.

You may find it challenging to make the switch from using the word "diet" to saying "nutrition." After all, we're inundated with marketing messages promoting weight loss that focus on "diet, diet, diet." If you don't believe me, go to any local bookstore, find the health and <u>diet</u> section, and almost every title includes the word "diet." "Why?" you might ask. That's an easy question to answer. Including the word "diet" in the title sells millions of books. People naturally associate the word "diet" with a cure or solution.

When I came up with the title of this book, "The Ah Ha's of Weight Loss," I purposely did not want the word "diet" in it. "Diet," to me, reflects a short-term approach to weight loss. I immediately hear "quick-start two-week diet," "the 10-week diet," "the 12-week diet," "the 'this' food diet" or "the 'that' food diet." You get the idea.

Ah Ha #10: Focus on Nutrition, Not on Diet

Say the word "diet" out loud. Doesn't it just sound short term with no real sense of permanence? Diet, to me, is about a short-term plan which is perhaps why 95% of all diets fail. If sustained weight-loss is your goal, you have to develop long-term habits. I trust that you not only want to lose the weight, but most importantly, you want to keep it off.

"Nutrition" is about a long-term, fuel-burning approach to weight loss. Remember, nutrition is your fuel. (See Ah Ha # 2.) Developing good nutritional habits enables you to make the right decisions, the right selections about the fuel that helps you go about your day-to-day life. The nutritional value that is in the fuel that you ingest determines not only your weight-loss, but your energy level, your confidence, and how you feel about learning more about health and fitness and pursuing that active lifestyle.

In fact, your awareness of what is nutritious and what is not will also help you enjoy occasional treats if you're upfront and honest with yourself. Knowing that you are deliberately choosing to eat or drink something that you know has literally no nutritional value can be rather empowering. You are deliberately choosing to eat the treat. You aren't sneaking it or fooling yourself into thinking it is anything else. You're empowered because you are in control.

Remember, think about nutrition and not diet. It may be viewed as semantics to most. However, the moment you start thinking about nutrition instead of diet, you're already way ahead on the pathway toward achieving a sustainable, healthy lifestyle.

You have a lifetime to achieve and maintain your weight loss goals. Stop torturing yourself with the unlikely results a quick-fix diet is claiming to provide. It's not about six, ten, or twelve weeks. It's about a lifetime of healthy living. Focus on nutrition, and you will find yourself looking at food in a whole new way.

You and the Mirror

1. Write down all the things you associate with the word "diet."

2. Write down all the things you associate with the word "nutrition."

3. Google the word "diet" and "nutrition" separately and compare results. Write down your perceived differences in the results. Which one feels more permanent and why?

Ah Ha #11: Never Skip Breakfast

I owe this Ah Ha to my wife. Thank you, Honey! At the peak of wanting to do something positive to impact my physical health, I unintentionally started doing more of the wrong things. Because of job pressures, I convinced myself that I could save time and calories by not eating breakfast. Then to make matters worse, I wouldn't eat lunch until 2:00 or 3:00 in the afternoon. Since I hadn't eaten breakfast or a morning snack, I'd consume a far bigger lunch than I should have.

I was constantly questioning myself: "I'm only eating two meals during the day, so how could I possibly be gaining weight?" What my wife Susan helped me realize is that by skipping breakfast and eating lunch later in the day, I was essentially putting my personal metabolism into hibernation. I wasn't fueling my body so that it could burn calories efficiently.

With her guidance, I finally started to connect the weight loss and nutrition dots. I figured out that I needed to spark my metabolism regularly, instead of just twice a day. I needed to keep adding fuel to my body so that I could continually burn calories. In addition to watching the number of calories I was consuming and keeping track of what I was eating, I needed to pay more attention to when I was eating as well.

Virtually all experts recommend that we eat five or six smaller meals throughout the day. The only way to get the metabolic process going is by eating something.

You might wonder then why so many people skip breakfast. Simple life pressures that consume our time and resources, such as working, raising kids and paying bills, get in the way. Skipping breakfast seems like a logical time-saver and a way to cut down on the number of calories consumed, but it couldn't be farther from the truth. When I hear people complain about their weight, the first question I often ask them is, "Do you eat breakfast?" Almost unanimously, the answer is either "no" or "sometimes" which continues to prove the important relationship between eating breakfast and losing weight. (By the way, although I'm a big fan, coffee isn't breakfast.)

For many people, skipping breakfast is a significant road block to losing weight. As an example, my mother-in-law, who lives locally and comes out to visit our girls regularly, gave me permission to tell her weight-loss-frustration story. Her previous job required her to put in long hours (7:00 a.m. until 9:00 p.m.) at an incredibly demanding job working in the West Wing of the White House. Partly because of all of the demands on her time and her desire to cut down on the calories consumed each day, she skipped breakfast. Now that she's taken a new position working 3 days per week, she frequently mentions her frustration about not being able to lose weight. However, when my wife and I ask her a basic question such as, "Did you eat breakfast this morning?" the answer is often, "No, not yet." When she does eat breakfast it's usually later in the morning around 9:30 or 10:00 am. The problem with this approach is that she's been up since 6:30 am so she's eating breakfast when she should really be eating her morning snack. Now that she has the time to eat breakfast, and she knows that she should, she still isn't doing it on a consistent basis or within the recommended one hour after she wakes up. This perceived insignificant habit is having a major negative impact on her weight loss goals.

Realize that my mother-in-law successfully raised five kids and maintained a professional career for over 20 years in high clearance government jobs, and yet she isn't connecting the fitness and nutrition dots either. If people like my mother-in-law aren't willing or knowledgeable enough to actually step back and evaluate their own habits with the intent of changing the harmful ones, how are people with far less of a support system than she has going to get it?

Ok, I hear some of you breakfast-skippers fighting me on this and shouting out the #1 excuse: "But I don't have enough time to eat breakfast!" If you have a commute, then you have time to eat at least a healthy nutrition bar while you're in the car. Or, you could buy an egg sandwich that is available just about anywhere, at food stands at the train station or the airport or near your office. It comes down to simply planning ahead and being prepared. Go with a convenient option, and if at all possible, make your breakfast choice a nutritious one as well.

Often times, I could easily skip breakfast if I didn't value its importance. I remember one morning, for example, that I had to catch a 6:00 a.m. train. I got up at 5:00 a.m. and left the house at 5:20. I was rushed, but I didn't skip breakfast. Instead, I built into my plan exactly where I was going to stop to get my egg sandwich and coffee. I still had my breakfast and actually got my metabolism started earlier than normal. Was the egg sandwich as nutritious as maybe low fat yogurt and granola? Probably not. It was a great source of protein, however, so my hunger was satisfied and I was able to stick to my routine of five small meals throughout the day.

Take the extra ten minutes in the morning to eat something. Eating most anything is better than eating nothing. Keep it simple with a bowl of whole grain cereal or a piece of toast with peanut butter. Or perhaps choose fresh fruit with yogurt or an egg sandwich.

I'm a big fan of high fiber and whole grains. They make me feel full and help my system stay regular. For example, a cereal containing six grams of fiber provides about 25% of the USDA daily recommended allowance. I like to consume 30 grams of fiber each day, so if I have one or two servings of cereal, I've already consumed almost half of my fiber goal in my first meal of the day. Some very simple high fiber choices include fruit, whole grain cereal or nutrition bars, and wheat toast with peanut butter.

Stop psyching yourself out by thinking that breakfast needs to be elaborate or that you need to vary what you eat for breakfast every day. Keep it convenient and simple. Breakfast should be the easiest meal of the day in terms of time and preparation. Think about it, even if you eat a doughnut or pancakes, at least it gets your metabolism started and you'll have all day to burn it off.

Remember, the metabolic process starts with food consumption. If you are not currently eating a healthy breakfast every day of the week including the weekends, you're really handicapping your weight loss efforts. Eating breakfast should be a significant priority. It's one of those "smarter-not-harder" pieces of advice, so I hope you learn from my mistakes.

Now that I'm maintaining rather than trying to lose weight, having a balanced breakfast remains a critical start to my day. It gets me going with my fuel and nutrition, and revs me up mentally as well. Eating breakfast creates an imaginary starting line for your nutrition awareness every single day, and the best part is, you don't even have to break a sweat to see the results!

You and the Mirror

1. How many times have you eaten breakfast in the past seven days?

2. From the time you get up in the morning, how many minutes pass until you eat breakfast? (Nutritional experts recommend eating within 1 hour of waking up.)

3. List below exactly what you ate for breakfast today:

4. If you don't eat breakfast daily, list the reasons why you don't:

5. If you do eat breakfast every day, list the benefits you gain by doing so:

6. List below what you plan to eat for breakfast tomorrow and what time you will enjoy it:

Ah Ha #12: Never Say "Never"

What is the best way to get someone to crave something? Tell them they can NEVER have it. Even if they didn't want it initially, now that you've told them they can't have it, they'll want it. That's human nature. If you don't believe me, just test this theory on any three-year-old and let me know how it goes.

In my research, strictly as a consumer, I have been encouraged to find that most industry professionals, whether they are trainers, nutritionists or diet authors, agree that you should never totally and consciously eliminate a favorite food.

Hundreds, if not thousands, of diets and eating regimens claim to help you lose weight. However, most don't focus on a realistic sustainable approach because they deny you from eating certain foods.

On the surface, it may seem counter intuitive that it's better to allow people to eat their favorite foods instead of eliminating these foods because they may not be good for their diet. If the goal is sustainable weight loss and maintenance and not the next fad diet, it is better to just limit the candy bar, pizza, jelly doughnut, (insert your weakness here) rather then trying to do without them completely. The overwhelming sentiment is that telling yourself "never" is not a sustainable strategy. If you try to deny yourself of your favorite foods, you're more likely to rebound and abuse that food item even more in the future. Perhaps this is a significant contributing factor as to why 95% of all diets fail and 75% of the dieters end up gaining more weight than when they started.

Armed with this comforting logical approach, I now fully subscribe to this theory. As an example, pizza is a family favorite in our house. Instead of eliminating it because it tends to be high in fat and calories and low in fiber, we've learned how to include it legitimately in our food regimen.

Case in point, we used to polish off a large pizza almost religiously every Friday night, which we realized wasn't a good idea considering my desire to eat healthfully and to lose weight. We decided to make a change without completely eliminating pizza from our regimen. First, we cut back on the frequency of our pizza consumption to about every third or fourth Friday. We also switched from a large to a medium pizza and added a salad to the meal.

I didn't have to deprive myself of pizza, yet without really thinking about it, I reduced my consumption from four pieces to two while adding some healthy raw vegetables from the salad. As this example demonstrates, you can use both portion size *and* frequency as levers to help you limit these foods without having to say goodbye to them forever.

Controlling portion size is a great way to improve your weight loss efforts. (More about portion control in Ah Ha #15). Our natural tendency is to grab the biggest portion just because that's what is normally served. Next time, consider going for a smaller portion of the same food to satisfy the craving without giving way to huge chunks of calories. Or, eat only half of what is normally served and box up the rest for another meal.

Here's another example of how to accommodate favorite foods into your food regimen. My wife loves chocolate. She confesses that she's incapable of having just one of something chocolate. As a result, she admits to overindulging on certain occasions. She then found a Hershey's 100 calorie dark chocolate bar that she eats almost nightly as her dessert. It fills her up, satisfies the chocolate craving and preserves her calorie count. It's a great alternative. I would also argue that her eating chocolate daily and incorporating it into her regular routine has diminished the pent-up desire to eat chocolate that she might have associated with it previously.

Amazingly, the food you perhaps once thought you couldn't live without becomes less important when you allow yourself to have it. What's more, having your clothes fit better and getting a few compliments from friends, neighbors and co-workers fuels the motivation to de-emphasize that food weakness. You build the momentum toward achieving even more success.

With the right balance of exercise and nutritional eating, you'll never have to say "never." In fact, depending on your commitment to yourself, you may even elect to eliminate a certain food just because it has lost its taste or usefulness. Now wouldn't that be progress!

You and the Mirror

1. What is your number #1 food weakness (a food that really isn't good for you that you don't think you can live without)?

2. What is your # 1 liquid weakness?

3. How often do you consume them?

    a. Food _____

    b. Liquid _____

4. Commit to a new schedule that reduces the frequency of these items:

    a. Next 7 days — 75% of current frequency.

    _____ number of times you'll consume your food weakness in the next 7 days.

    _____ number of times you'll consume your liquid weakness in the next 7 days.

    b. Days 8–20 — 50% of current frequency.

    _____ number of times you'll consume your food weakness in the next 8-20 days.

    _____ number of times you'll consume your liquid weakness in the next 8-20 days.

c. Days 21 and beyond — 25% of current frequency.

_____ number of times you'll consume your food weakness in the next 21 days and beyond.

_____ number of times you'll consume your liquid weakness in the next 21 days and beyond.

Ah Ha #13: Wasted Calories — Liquids

Stealing back wasted calories by modifying your liquid consumption is actually quite easy. This is a good example of how making slight modifications to what you consume can make a big difference. You may even find that doing so won't even require you to make huge sacrifices.

Below are the nutritional labels for some popular thirst quenchers. Have fun with this as you try to match the label with its brand.

A

Nutrition Facts
Serving Size 1 cup (8 oz.)
Servings Per Container about 2

Amount Per Serving

Calories 130 — Calories from Fat 0

Total Fat 0g
    Saturated Fat 0g
    Trans Fat 0g
Cholesterol mg
Sodium 35 mg
Total Carbohydrate 33g
    Dietary Fiber 0g
    Sugars 33g
Protein 0g

B

Nutrition Facts
Serving Size 1 cup (8 oz.)
Servings Per Container 2.5

Amount Per Serving

Calories 50 — Calories from Fat 0

Total Fat 0g
    Saturated Fat 0g
    Trans Fat 0g
Cholesterol mg
Sodium 110mg
Total Carbohydrate 14g
    Dietary Fiber 0g
    Sugars 14g
Protein 0g

Ah Ha #13: Wasted Calories — Liquids

Nutrition Facts
Serving Size 1 cup (8 oz.)
Servings Per Container 2.5

Amount Per Serving
Calories 40   Calories from Fat 0

Total Fat 0g
　Saturated Fat 0g
　Trans Fat 0g
Cholesterol   mg
Sodium 20 mg
Total Carbohydrate 16g
　Dietary Fiber 0g
　Sugars 10g
Protein 0g

C

Nutrition Facts
Serving Size 1 cup (8 oz.)
Servings Per Container about 2

Amount Per Serving
Calories 60   Calories from Fat 0

Total Fat 0g
　Saturated Fat 0g
　Trans Fat 0g
Cholesterol   mg
Sodium 0 mg
Total Carbohydrate 15g
　Dietary Fiber 0g
　Sugars 15g
Protein 0g

D

Nutrition Facts
Serving Size 1 cup (8 oz.)
Servings Per Container 2.5

Amount Per Serving
Calories 50   Calories from Fat 0

Total Fat 0g
　Saturated Fat 0g
　Trans Fat 0g
Cholesterol   mg
Sodium 0 mg
Total Carbohydrate 13g
　Dietary Fiber 0g
　Sugars 13g
Protein 0g

E

Nutrition Facts
Serving Size 1 cup (8 oz.)
Servings Per Container 2.5

Amount Per Serving
Calories 100   Calories from Fat 0

Total Fat 0g
　Saturated Fat 0g
　Trans Fat 0g
Cholesterol   mg
Sodium 35 mg
Total Carbohydrate 27g
　Dietary Fiber 0g
　Sugars 27g
Protein 0g

F

The Ah Ha's of Weight Loss

____ Snapple Green Tea

____ Coca-Cola

____ Life Water Agave Lemonade

____ Gatorade Orange

____ Ocean Spray Cranberry Juice

____ Vitamin Water Kiwi Strawberry

*Answers on last page of chapter

No doubt you noticed the major discrepancy in calories among these varieties of common drinks. Take a good hard look at the number of calories in a regular soda vs. a diet soda. Attention regular soda drinkers—do me a favor and just try to swap your regular sodas with diet sodas for a specified period of time, say seven days. I know, I just heard the moans. But give it a try. I think you'll be surprised that today's diet sodas are not nearly as bad-tasting as they used to be due to the advancement of no-calorie sweeteners. Of course, the best option is to drink only water. Realistically, drinking only water isn't something I can do, but I certainly encourage you to do so if you can.

Now let's look at other wasted calories in liquids—those early morning thirst quenchers and frozen morning drinks that seem to be popping up at every major fast food chain from McDonald's to Dunkin' Donuts to Starbucks. If you start your day with one of these and call it breakfast, you're cheating yourself. If you can't live without these calorie-laden behemoths, then put them on your just-every-once-in-a-while rotation and consider them a treat rather than a staple. The fact is that some of these early morning refreshers have upwards of 1000 calories or almost 50% of your recommended daily intake.

You and I don't need a Ph.D. to realize that consuming over half your calories when your day is just getting started seems out of balance. Ideally, you should cut out these drinks, or at a minimum, you should modify them with either non-fat options if offered, get the smallest size available or drastically limit their frequency.

Let's take a peek at the menu of the country's most recognized coffee brand. Do you realize that a Starbuck's vente (large) Mint Mocha Chip Frappuccino® blended coffee with Chocolate Whipped Cream has 590 calories? If you get it without whipped cream, it's 460 calories, or a tall (small—a paltry 12 ounces) has 360 calories with whipped cream and 270 without. Just by ordering the smallest size and eliminating the whipped cream, you can save a whopping 320 calories! If you made this one small change yet still drank one every weekday, you would be saving 83,200 calories per year which translates into almost 24 pounds!

Let's see what happens if you switch to their light blended version of the same beverage—a Starbuck's Mint Mocha Chip Frappuccino® Light Blended Coffee vente (large) without whipped cream has 310 calories and a tall (small) only has 170. If you just can't do without a mint mocha chip frappuccino, simply by choosing the light blended version, you can make a huge impact in your calorie consumption for that one beverage. For this example let's look at the opportunity to cut down on calories over the course of a year—that's a savings of an additional 100 calories per day over 5 days each week for 52 weeks bringing the grand total to an additional 26,000 fewer calories. Drum roll please…or that adds up to another 7 pounds! That's right, I just showed you how to maintain your indulgence *and* lose 31 pounds in the process. This, my friends, is real weight loss for real people, and it only requires that you make one tiny little adjustment.

Just as important if you are trying to lose weight is acknowledging the negative caloric impact alcohol has on your goals. You're fairly safe with most light beers coming in around the 100 calorie mark, but if you have two or three of them, the calories can add up fast.

The cocktails listed on the enticing exotic drink menu are the ones to be weary of. Those tantalizing marketing masterpieces resting on the table often include beverages that have over 200 calories per drink because they contain fruit juice or some high calorie mixers that are loaded with sugar. Sure, they taste good, but I would steer clear of them entirely, at least until you've achieved your goal weight.

A great alternative to high calorie drinks that still taste great are the powdered mixes for water such as Crystal Light. These are incredibly convenient and come in multiple flavors, but they only have 5–15 calories per serving or bottle size mix. I think these are a fantastic alternative and will likely get you to drink more water which is a great goal.

Eighty percent of your body is made up of water. Staying hydrated is important to your overall health. You need to keep replenishing your fluids. So drink up…but choose wisely. The calories saved could be your own.

You and the Mirror

1. List all the liquids you drank today and the calories in each one.

   Beverage _____   Calories _____

   Beverage _____   Calories _____

   Beverage _____   Calories _____

   Beverage _____   Calories _____

   Beverage _____   Calories _____

   Beverage _____   Calories _____

2. List below the number of ounces of water you drank today.

   _____ ounces of water

3. List some alternatives to the higher calorie beverages you consume.

   High calorie beverage _____

   Possible substitute _____

   High calorie beverage _____

   Possible substitute _____

   High calorie beverage _____

   Possible substitute _____

High calorie beverage _____

Possible substitute _____

High calorie beverage _____

Possible substitute _____

Answers to Beverage Labels

- D Snapple Green Tea
- F Coca-Cola
- C Life Water Agave Lemonade
- B Gatorade Orange
- A Ocean Spray Cranberry Juice
- E Vitamin Water Kiwi Strawberry

Ah Ha #14: Nutrition Labels 101

A few chapters back I promised to go over nutrition labels in more detail, so here we go. Although nutrition labels were designed to place knowledge into the hands of the consumer, they aren't completely straight forward and can sometimes be misleading. Two of the most troubling numbers on the labels are servings per container and serving size.

First, let's consider servings per container. It is easy to mistakenly think the nutrition items delineated on the label represent the values for the contents of the entire container you are holding in your hand. It is very easy to look only at the nutritional content and count the values listed accordingly without noticing the number of servings in the container. What often trips most people up, including me when I first started my weight loss and fitness journey, is that many times the servings-per-container are more than one. Let's take a look at some everyday food items. Note the number of servings per container in each product.

The Ah Ha's of Weight Loss

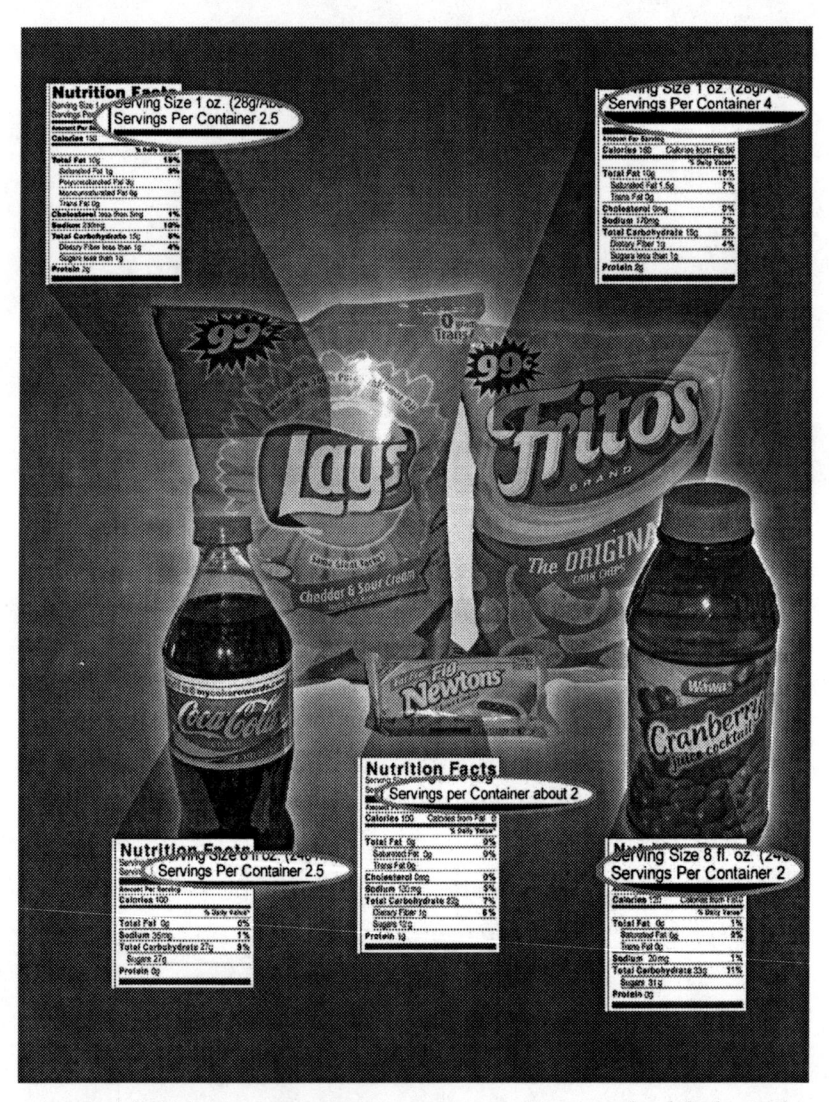

Now let's look at calories per serving. Notice the label on the bag of Lay's chips. The bag in the illustration contains 2.5 servings at 150 calories per serving, a total of 375 calories for the entire bag. Who in their right mind is only going to eat 15 of the total number of chips included in the "single" bag? If you just glance at the label and see 150 calories, you might think, "That's not bad" without realizing that there are really 2.5 servings in the bag. Before you know it, you've eaten the whole bag of chips down to those last few

98

Ah Ha #14: Nutrition Labels 101

miniscule crumbs that you dig out of the crevices in the bottom of the bag. That means you just consumed 375 calories instead of the 150 you thought you were consuming.

Now look at the bag of Fritos corn chips. For the record, I've got nothing against Fritos and actually ate them as a kid, but let's scrutinize those numbers on the label. First of all, the actual bag of corn chips is dimensionally smaller than the bag of regular chips, so subconsciously you might be thinking that since the bag is smaller, the number of calories must be in the acceptable range for a snack. Then, if you flip the bag over, you notice there are a surprising four servings in this one bag that we both know will be polished off with your sandwich. That means that when you multiply 160 calories x 4 servings you'd consume a whopping 640 calories in one lousy bag. I know from experience that a lot of people would have seen the 160 calories for the corn chips and compared it to the 150 calories in the regular chips and said to themselves, "It's only another 10 calories." So be careful! Some of these manufacturers trick you because the stats on the nutrition label seem reasonable until you look at corresponding serving size.

Another major culprit in this game of nutrition label confusion is fruit juices and sodas. We just learned in Ah Ha #13 how your favorite drink can really be harming your weight loss progress without you even realizing it. We also learned about the wide variance in calories for the same basic Starbucks drink depending on size and ingredients. Now, let's take a look at the most popular drink in the world, a bottle of Coke. It contains 2.5 servings—not 2, not 3, but the odd number of two-and-a-half. Again, it's highly unlikely that most of us would be able to drink just 8 ounces of the 20 ounces in a single bottle of Coke. With the configuration of the bottle, short of weighing the amount you intend to drink, it would be difficult to know exactly how much of the bottle would equal 8 ounces anyway. Or worse yet, you might fall victim to my old excuse when I would say to myself, "I don't want to waste it." Glug, glug, glug, AHHHH.

My primary point is to make sure you look closely at the number of servings and do the appropriate math to ensure you truly understand the calorie impact of what you are consuming. This sounds so simple, but packaging logic and nutritional logic might not always match up, so consumer beware—figure out serving size and calories per serving before you indulge .

To be fair, Coke at least does the math for you in an effort to educate you on how many total calories are included in one bottle of soda. It's scary to think that many people drink more than one bottle of soda each day. If a regular bottle of Coke contains 250 calories, and you drink two per day, that means that 25% of your recommended daily 2,000 calorie intake (500 calories) is accounted for. The worst part is that it provides virtually no nutritional value.

Now let's look at other items on the nutrition label that are important in managing your weight, specifically calories, fat grams, carbohydrates, fiber and protein. These are the items you should understand first as you build your knowledge about nutrition.

First, calories —as discussed earlier in this book, it is critical to understand the caloric value of the food you are consuming. The number of calories you consume is the absolute most important metric to understand as it directly relates to losing weight. As you'll recall, if you consume more calories than your body uses, you will gain weight. Conversely, to lose weight you have to burn more calories than you consume. So initially, when you're trying to understand the nutrition label, focus on calories. Once you've mastered your understanding of calorie intake, you're then ready to move on to increase your understanding of other important items on the nutrition label and what they mean to your weight loss efforts.

Calories from fat is also an important indicator. Most experts recommend that you limit fat intake to about 30% of the calories you eat. However, read labels carefully on items marked "low fat" and "no fat." Many of these items are loaded with calories which sounds contradictory. Focusing too heavily on eating no fat and low fat foods that may be deceivingly loaded with calories may sabotage your weight loss efforts and fool you into thinking that you're making good choices. In reality these items may be sending you down a negative path on your weight loss journey.

Fat is actually an important nutrient that your body uses for growth and development. By no means do you want to eliminate fat from your regimen. You just want to be careful to limit fat consumption to no more than 30% of your daily caloric intake.

Next, carbohydrates and fiber—much debate occurs about whether carbohydrates are good or bad for you. In spite of what some diet programs claim, carbs are not the enemy. Carbs are your body's primary source of energy. Fiber and sugar are types of carbohydrates. Healthy sources, like fruits, vegetables, yogurt, beans, and whole grains, can reduce the risk of heart disease and improve digestive functioning.

When it comes to the nutrition label relative to carbs and fiber, read the information carefully. Aim for carbs that are high in fiber and stay away from those with added sugar such as sodas, cakes, pastries, sweetened cereals and candy which only add calories without adding many nutrients.

It's no secret that I'm a believer in moderation. Include carbohydrates in your regimen, but don't overdo it! Some carbs are not only good for you, but they can help you lose weight, especially if you choose the carbs that are also high in fiber. If an item has 20 grams of carbs and 6 grams of fiber, then the real number of net carbs is 14 not 20. Fiber is a subset of the total grams of carbohydrates. Fiber is a critical component to one's diet, and yet many people don't eat enough of it. Fiber not only helps your digestive system, but it also provides a fullness factor that makes you feel full and reduces your appetite.

Finally, protein—Your body needs protein to build and repair essential parts of the body, such as muscles, blood, and organs. Choose proteins that are lean (low in fat) and low in cholesterol, such as chicken, fish, and lean meats. Personally, I strive for a high fiber and high protein regimen.

Be patient. When it comes to truly understanding nutrition, no shortcut or instant gratification here. Take time to learn the fundamentals before moving on to the finer details on the nutrition label. After all, you wouldn't think of adding a second floor or an addition to your house until you have finished the foundation. Take time to master the basics on the nutrition label before you get concerned about the minor items.

So many people try to get too sophisticated with the nutrition knowledge. For example, they try to figure out what foods they should be eating together for maximum efficiency. Or, they are concerned about which day they should eat fish versus lean meat and whether or not the vegetables should be raw or cooked and complemented with a warm or cold beverage. Who cares! That's well above what most people need to understand or worry about and just compounds the confusion. Remember, if it's too complex or cumbersome, you won't stick with it which will only lead to more frustration.

We see this all the time with exercise to prove my point. Many people try to leap frog to more complex fitness rather than mastering the basics first. A common question I hear often is, *"Should I work out in the morning, afternoon or evening?"* The answer: just work out—period, regardless of when you do it. Quite simply, work out when you know you can stick to a game plan that translates into consistency. If you're somebody who is not going to ever be up at 5:00 a.m., don't sign up for a 5:00 a.m. boot-camp class. You're setting yourself up to fail. Is there scientific evidence that states you should exercise at an optimum time of the day? Maybe. That's not my concern. My concern is to build that foundation of consistency which means setting yourself up for success.

Keep it simple. Concentrate on knowing how to read a nutrition label appropriately and understanding your total calorie consumption. Start leveraging the right food groups in your regimen on a consistent basis. Once you've mastered the basics, then feel free to move on to the more complex items.

Eat the right foods, choose fruits and vegetables, and you can't go wrong. The goal is to build baseline rules and knowledge—the foundation—so you can build confidence and decide to learn more in the future if you want. Concentrate on building the baseline knowledge you need to lead an active, healthy and fulfilling life. That's the goal, after all, isn't it?

You and the Mirror

1. Cut out and paste below the nutrition labels from three items you ate today. Beside the label, note anything special or especially helpful information on the label, such as "good high fiber, low fat option"; or "be careful—container has 4 servings," etc.

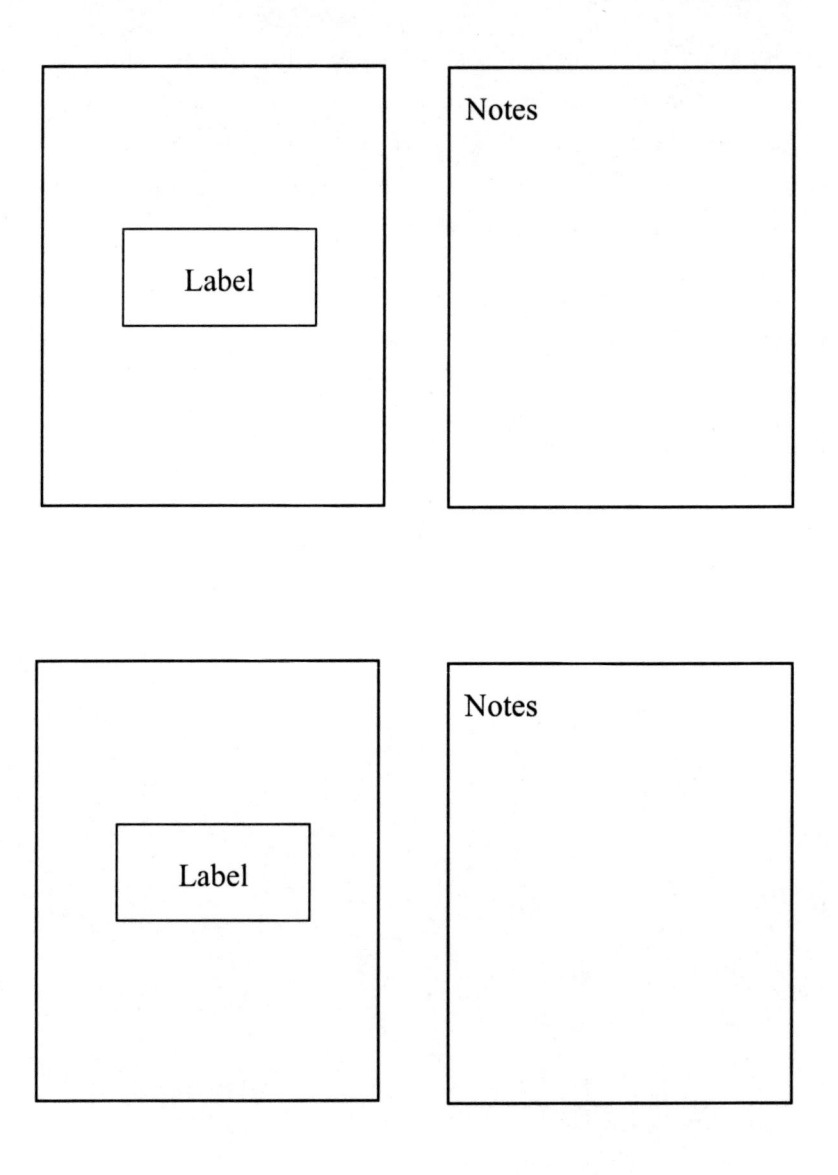

Label	Notes
Label	Notes

Ah Ha #14: Nutrition Labels 101

```
┌─────────────────┐   ┌─────────────────┐
│                 │   │ Notes           │
│                 │   │                 │
│    ┌───────┐    │   │                 │
│    │ Label │    │   │                 │
│    └───────┘    │   │                 │
│                 │   │                 │
│                 │   │                 │
└─────────────────┘   └─────────────────┘
```

Read the nutrition label on everything you consume today. (don't forget sauces, dressings, condiments, etc.) Did anything surprise you when you read these labels?

ITEM   SURPRISES

_____   _____

_____   _____

_____   _____

_____   _____

_____   _____

_____   _____

_____   _____

_____   _____

Ah Ha #15: Portion Control Means Gaining Control

News flash! You don't have to eat the hungry-man portion of food on your oversized plate just because it was served to you. Use logic and common sense when it comes to determining the portions you will consume and how often you will eat.

I personally subscribe to a meal plan that includes eating small portions frequently, including breakfast, late morning snack, lunch, afternoon snack and dinner. This plan keeps my metabolism engaged throughout the day and prevents me from being ravenous for the next meal. It allows me to feel fuller and fends off any cravings. This plan works even better when I select foods that are higher in fiber combined with more protein-enriched foods which naturally make me feel fuller.

If you don't have a handle on portion control, the caloric intake part of the calories-consumed-vs.-calories-burned equation is going to be more challenging. If you feel the need to simply eat more, make a bigger salad or load up on an extra portion of veggies. At least be smart enough to realize the danger of overindulging if your portions are beginning to overflow the plate.

Isn't it odd that when you eat out, restaurants naturally tend to give you overflowing portions of everything? They package the daily specials or offer food items in combination platters with an abundance of extra sides. Perhaps, it's to build value and to make you think you're getting more for your money. Don't fall prey to this trap! Just order what you truly want and don't feel pressured to get the combo just because the items are bundled that way.

One day, for breakfast at a restaurant in New York City I ordered two eggs, no home fries, bacon and toast. (That's often what I'll order when I go out for breakfast.) The waitress looked at me funny and said, "It comes with three eggs and potatoes." I knew this because it was well described on the menu, so I politely said, "But, I only want two eggs and no potatoes." She paused again and said, "Well, it comes with three." I said, "You can charge me for three, but I only want to eat two eggs, so you can save the extra egg for the next customer." She reluctantly agreed and was probably thinking I was cheating myself by not getting something I was paying for. To her defense, two out of three U.S. adults aren't overweight or obese because they turned down items already included with a meal on the menu. If it's included, most people take it, and usually eat it, even though they may not want it or need it. It might have actually been the first time she had a customer ask for less food. I think it's a telling story and rather indicative of our society whereby we're almost being forced to eat.

Similarly, when you order any sandwich or hamburger, what's the usual side order that comes with it? French fries. Do you have to eat them? Well, of course not, but you probably will eat them because they have been served to you. Let's be honest, it's tough to stare down a mound of tempting French fries without at least nibbling on a few of them. As an alternative, I encourage you to take a more active role in your ordering experience. Consider requesting a side of fruit, or ask what other sides they have to offer. If it's not a food that appeals to you, just ask that it be omitted. If the hamburger shows up with the fries, don't expect that your will-power will be strong enough to resist eating them. Chances are you'll give in and eat them just because they're there. Send your order back and ask them to remove the French fries.

I used to eat fries with every meal, simply because they were served to me, even though I hadn't specified them when I ordered. For many casual dining restaurants, the main course or sandwich just naturally came with them. Now I ask for other side dishes instead and only eat fries maybe once a month. I'm aware of what the side dishes are that come with the main course, and I don't hesitate to request a replacement: side salad, side of fruit or vegetables or perhaps nothing. Yes, you can even decline food items even though they come with the meal. That's your right as the customer.

Ok, so now you're empowered. The next time you go out to eat and a food item comes with something you just don't want to eat, or you're going to be tempted to eat it, ask for a substitute. It's that easy. Same goes for portion control. If you know the portions are going to be huge, here are some easy options: Don't order it, order a smaller size, split it with a spouse or friend, get an appetizer instead, order a kid's portion, or manage the portion by leaving some behind. Another option is to request a "to-go" box as soon as your oversized order is served, and before even tasting it, pack half of it to take home to enjoy for lunch or dinner the next day or two. Remember, you are not obligated to be a member of the "clean-plate" club.

Most of the focus on portion control has been on servings at restaurants. The reason is that we're eating out more and more often, and that's when we seem to face the biggest portion-control challenges. Portion control is equally important at home. Don't be afraid to freeze meat, poultry and fish as opposed to cooking it all just because that's the size you purchased from the grocery store. Also, pay attention to the number of servings in a recipe and divvy up your servings accordingly.

Ah Ha #15: Portion Control Means Gaining Control

Another often overlooked strategy to help get a better handle on portion control is speed of consumption. Basically "speed consumption" means the time it takes to eat and swallow the food on your plate. Personally, I still struggle with this and know I eat way too fast. By eating too quickly, we don't give our digestive system enough time to report back to our brain that we're full. By purposely taking a bite of food and putting down the fork and chewing the food to completion before taking the next bite, we can literally stretch a smaller portion of food longer. I'm envious of those like my 3-year-old daughter who is so deliberate with each bite. She chews it completely until every last morsel is swallowed before thinking about the next bite. She can literally take up to an hour to eat lunch or dinner. I need to constantly coach myself that eating slowly is a good thing when we live in a hurry-up world. She's a great role model for me in this regard and something I continually work to improve.

This Ah Ha about portion control sounds so simple, and it is. However, it really takes discipline and foresight to control portion size. When you are successful in controlling your portions, you can experience a renewed sense of confidence that stems from being in control. Simply take the few extra seconds to think about the size of an item and which sides are included. Taking control and deciding if you want to eat it can be very empowering.

You and the Mirror

1. The last time you ate at a restaurant, what sides did you eat with your meal?

   Were they a good choice? _____ yes _____ no

   If no, what other sides could you have ordered?

2. The last time you ate at home, what sides did you eat with your meal?

   Were they a good choice? _____ yes _____ no

   If no, what other sides could you have eaten?

3. List below the times you plan to eat tomorrow: (Goal: Eat small portions frequently.)

   Wake up _____

   Breakfast _____

   Snack _____

   Lunch _____

   Snack _____

   Dinner _____

   Bedtime _____

Ah Ha #16: If You Don't Want To Eat It, Don't Bring It Home

If you don't want to eat it, don't bring it home. Like many of the other Ah Ha's, it sounds so simple, and it is. Yet it's equally effective. Ask yourself, "When I do my own grocery shopping and I eat at home, am I more disciplined than if I'm on vacation and I eat at a restaurant every night?" Most of us will answer "yes." We are much more disciplined when we control our own environment. Since we acknowledge that we're more disciplined if we control our own environment, let's do just that.

Look around your pantry, cupboards, refrigerator, and freezer. Are there items in there you know you shouldn't be eating and, therefore, you should remove them immediately? Get rid of them. Don't set yourself up for failure. If you don't remove them, you will eat them, and you will feel guilty about eating them. You'll have the added mental struggle on top of the physical weight gain. Put another way, why would they even be in your kitchen if you didn't intend to eat them at some point? UHHH, exactly!

If there is a food item that you're going to be tempted to eat, trust me, I've been there, you're going to eat it. What you're first going to say is, "I'm only going to have one, half, a little or a bite." That then leads into, "Well, I don't want to throw it away and waste it, so let me just finish it." Or, "I'm buying this for my kids or spouse, and I'll just have a little bit." It never works. You're setting yourself up for failure. If you don't want to eat it, don't bring it into the house. It's that simple.

Have you ever rented a vacation house and made everyone responsible for purchasing a portion of the groceries? We recently did a week at the beach in the Outer Banks on the North Carolina coast with Susan's family. Everybody brought the fun food which included multiple styles of chips, dips, pretzels, crackers and various other munchies. I found myself eating items that I hadn't eaten in two years, just because they were around. That's what happens, especially when you're not constantly busy doing things you normally do. You get out of your normal routine. You see the chips. You're looking for something to do. Your guard is down, and you eat them. Now, I probably wouldn't have purchased those same chips at home, but because they're around the vacation house and I was hungry or bored, I ate them. The same philosophy applies at home or at work. If the items are around, you're going to eat them!

If you're still not convinced about the simple yet critical importance of this Ah Ha, tune in to any of the weight loss shows—whether it's The Biggest Loser or Dr. Oz or any number of TV specials that try to help people understand and change their habits with the goal of weight loss in mind. The first thing they do is raid the participant's personal kitchen. They literally go through the kitchen and haul out trash bags filled with less-than-nutritious foods. In some cases the family is left with virtually nothing in the cabinets because so much of their food was unhealthy. In fact, in one episode of a show, they actually had to bring in a small dumpster because the family had mounds upon mounds of unhealthy food in their home. It was obviously entertaining, but really made me think about how toxic our own "safe" surroundings really can be.

Conversely, if you surround yourself with nutritious foods that are high in fiber, protein, and nutrients, then you'll eat those too

Ah Ha #16: If You Don't Want To Eat It, Don't Bring It Home

without giving it much thought. If you're really hungry and all you have to eat are nuts, fruit, vegetables, hummus and other things that are good for you, you're going to eat them.

Set yourself up for success. Surround yourself with foods that are good for you and will promote your weight loss efforts, and get rid of the rest.

I've never been a fan of trying to follow a rigid menu schedule—preset, full menus for every day of the week. When I look at those included in many of the popular magazines and weight loss programs, I don't see sustainability. The reality is, if the menu schedule is too rigid, then you're going to say, "It's taking too much time and effort to shop for the ingredients and prepare the meals," which elevates the stress level and generates negative energy into a topic that's supposed to be basic, sustainable and successful.

People eat according to their habits anyway. If you eat fish and chicken, the likelihood is you've probably fallen into a pattern where you eat them "x" number of times a week. If you were to look back at the last six months, you've probably established a pattern. If you have hamburgers once every couple of weeks, you'll probably continue to do the same. You establish a pattern of eating, and you tend to repeat that pattern over time, especially when you're eating at home.

Remember, keep the process of making food choices simple. First, read the nutrition label, understand it, and ask, "Is this good for me?" Next, make some general realizations about the main course, such as, "I need some more substantial items for dinner." This is where you can group items like chicken, fish, whole grain pasta and lean beef. Once you've decided on the main course, the next logical question is, "What are the things that I want to accompany it?" Consider some brown rice, salad, raw vegetables or steamed vegetables. Then you can create some regular snack food items and expand on those categories.

Another approach is to categorize your choices into breakfast items, morning and afternoon snacks, lunch items, and dinner items. Don't be rigid in your choices. Be flexible while still maintaining control.

In our often hectic lives of juggling work, family and activities, I think it's unrealistic to say, "Next Tuesday, I'm going to have chicken cacciatore, with a side medley of steamed vegetables, and six ounces of milk." That, to me, sounds like too much work. Again, I encourage general planning, but don't over do it. If you're too rigid, what will likely happen is that you'll miss a scheduled meal, get down on yourself and then the negative thoughts will take over. Keep it simple and manage the categories so that they are interchangeable and easy to prepare.

Ah Ha #16: If You Don't Want To Eat It, Don't Bring It Home

You and the Mirror

1. Take inventory in your cabinets and fridge and remove items that you feel are high in calories and low in nutritional value. List below the items that you removed:

   _____   _____

   _____   _____

   _____   _____

   _____   _____

   _____   _____

2. Remove all items in your home that contain HFCS (high fructose corn syrup) or enriched white flour within the first 5 ingredients listed on the package. List below the items that you removed:

   _____   _____

   _____   _____

   _____   _____

   _____   _____

   _____   _____

3. What percentage of your food currently in your home is fresh vs. processed?

   Fresh   _____%

   Processed   _____%

The Ah Ha's of Weight Loss

4. For the next 24 hours, attempt to eat only whole grains and natural foods. List below the whole grains and natural foods you ate during that time period:

_____   _____

_____   _____

_____   _____

_____   _____

_____

Ah Ha #17: You Can't Reach a Goal Tomorrow If You Don't Know Where You Are Today

Ask anyone who has ever worked for me, and they'll tell you that this Ah Ha is one of my favorites. I firmly believe that in order to reach your goal tomorrow, you have to know where you are today—your starting point, if you will.

Prior to creating JumpSnap, I was in sales management and have participated in every facet of sales throughout my career. The one thing I love most about sales people is that they are almost always positive. They use terms like "great" and "fantastic" and "excellent" to describe how they're doing and feeling. While I love these positive adjectives, they simply don't work when referring to goals. How do you measure "great"? For one person "great" could be accomplishing 20% of a goal and to another it could be achieving 200% of a goal.

Let's keep it simple, remove the emotion and focus on the facts. If your goal is 20 sales per day and you've only achieved 10 sales, then I'm not sure what's so "great" about your accomplishment. Now I'm not one of those hard-nosed bosses who never gives positive feedback, quite the opposite in fact. However, I do spend a lot of time challenging people to take the emotion out of goal setting and stick to the facts. The same concept applies to setting your own health and fitness goals.

When you set goals, it's imperative to know where you are today and map out where you want to end up. I've found that it's often easier and much more tangible to work backwards from your end goal. For example, I originally wanted to end up at 175 pounds. In years past I would pick random dates from the calendar by which I wanted to achieve my goals, thus violating one of my beliefs about the basics of goal setting. If I had followed my own advice and used the facts of my current weight at the time, I quickly would have realized I was setting myself up for failure because the math wasn't realistic.

After I realized I wasn't following my own belief, I took a step back and started mapping out a game plan. Using my personal example, at my heaviest I weighed about 205 lbs., so that meant I needed to lose 30 lbs. I started my workout in September 2004 and thought achieving my desired weight by my birthday of April 14, 2005 was a good goal. I figured that I had seven months or roughly four pounds per month, which translated into about one pound per week, to achieve my goal weight.

Now I know that doesn't sound terribly exciting, and seven months probably seems like an eternity. But remember, I was interested in sustained weight loss, and this approach was realistic.

To summarize my weight loss goal setting approach—start where you are (baseline), determine where you want to be (goal), and then set up a realistic plan to get you there.

To create a baseline, you have to understand where you are today. Most people know that they're overweight, but like me, they aren't willing to admit how far they've let themselves go. As much as you may dread doing so, you have to get on the scale to understand how overweight you are. If you've talked to anybody who set out on a track to lose the extra pounds that have crept up on them over the years, almost invariably, they will tell you they never knew how overweight they had become. They either avoided the scale or the

Ah Ha #17: You Can't Reach a Goal If You Don't Know Where You Are

mirror, or they just chose not to accept it. However, when they make that final commitment, they almost always say, "I never knew I had gotten that large," For whatever reason, people don't acknowledge the facts. You have to know where you're starting so you can set realistic goals in order to allow yourself the best opportunity to succeed.

As you work through your weight loss plan, you should be honest with yourself and recognize potential road blocks. For me, I realized that special occasions such as the holiday season would likely affect my goals, so I anticipated no weight loss those weeks. I know this approach is terribly boring and not very mysterious, but it's exactly how you gain real results. You've heard all the sayings "baby steps," "one game at a time," "chip away at it"—but they actually work.

I firmly believe you should write down your goals and document progress toward achieving them. That's one of the main reasons I decided to create the "You and the Mirror" section at the end of each Ah Ha. Don't just keep them in your head. If they're in your head, they're too easy to change or lose track of. If you write them down, you're making a visible commitment to yourself. With a written record of your goals, you can go back and review what you said you were going to do.

There will be days when you will exceed your goals and other days when you will fall short. If you have them in writing, you'll always have a benchmark you can go back to and measure your progress against. If your goals are just in your head, they're not real.

What I did in previous weight loss attempts prior to getting serious about losing weight was pick a day out of thin air and say, "I'm going to lose XX pounds by this date," which is foolish. I didn't do the simple math to make sure that my target date was even feasible. You have to be realistic, or you're merely setting yourself up to fail.

First, we need to recognize how we can achieve our goals. Start with the simple things. What's your current weight? What are you ingesting? What's your caloric intake for the items you're ingesting? Are you exercising? Just looking at weight, your exercise regime (if you have one), and what you're consuming is a great place to start. Then you can build your weight loss and fitness plan from there.

In my case, my goal was to lose 30 lbs. At that point, I weighed 205 lbs. I worked backwards from there to determine my timeline and plan for losing the 30 lbs. To get started, I kept a health and fitness diary. I couldn't just think about where I was, but I needed to know factually where I was.

Don't guess you're at 185 lbs. simply because you're unwilling to admit that you're really 205 lbs. You'll never get down to the weight that you really want that is sustainable and lifelong.

Did I mention 95% of all diets fail?

Results are the one thing that will guarantee you will stick to your plan. If people don't see results in the first few days, many of them quit. Quitting is often followed by an introspective and convincing, *"Well, it didn't work for me."* Well, the person didn't give it any time to work, so of course it wasn't going to work. Setting realistic goals will enable you to get through natural plateaus, which will allow you an opportunity to succeed before the quitting thoughts start entering your brain.

It takes time. Most people have been adding on the weight for years and years. Why would you expect it to be gone in just a couple of months? It's unrealistic. You have to be realistic.

We've talked a lot about exercise and about nutrition as the foundation for building healthy habits. Now, it's time to put it all together and allow it to work for you. Goal-setting is a critical component to leveraging your knowledge and turning it into results.

Ah Ha #17: You Can't Reach a Goal If You Don't Know Where You Are

You and the Mirror

1. How much do you weigh today?

2. What is your dream weight that would give you unstoppable confidence?

3. Subtract your current weight from your dream weight. This is how many weeks it should take you to achieve your goal. Write your goal weight date below:

4. Regardless of how many weeks or months into the future it might be, place your goal weight date on your calendar and commit to it. Track your progress below:

Starting weight _____ Goal weight date _____

End of Week 1   Current weight _____

End of Week 2   Current weight _____

End of Week 3   Current weight _____

End of Week 4   Current weight _____

End of Week 5   Current weight _____

End of Week 6   Current weight _____

End of Week 7   Current weight _____

End of Week 8   Current weight _____

The Ah Ha's of Weight Loss

End of Week 9   Current weight _____

End of Week 10   Current weight _____

End of Week 11   Current weight _____

End of Week 12   Current weight _____

End of Week 13   Current weight _____

End of Week 14   Current weight _____

End of Week 15   Current weight _____

End of Week 16   Current weight _____

Ah Ha #18: How to Measure Success

The scale can be a scary reminder of how we've let ourselves go. Yet, it can be a powerful tool that builds immense confidence when you begin to see the numbers drop.

Some say that you shouldn't get on a scale because the numbers can be discouraging. If you begin a new workout and the scale doesn't reflect any weight loss immediately, yes, you may get frustrated and be tempted to quit. But I say, you need to use the scale to take advantage of what it has to tell you. View it as a tool that measures your success, or for that matter, identifies your opportunity for improvement. The scale is, after all, the best way to determine if you need to lose weight.

Please don't be one of those people who gets on the scale, doesn't like the numbers and rationalizes why it's not telling the real story. You know what they say, "This scale must be broken." "It's probably water weight." "I'm sure I'll weigh less in the morning." If you're overweight, the hard truth is that you're simply not healthy regardless of what you try to tell yourself. Sure, you might not be suffering any immediate side effects from your excess weight today, but you will.

In addition to watching my numbers drop on the scale, I found great comfort in how my clothes fit as I started to lose weight. As mentioned previously, the telling moment that drove me to change my habits was when I realized that my size 36 inch waist pants were getting extremely tight. To get them on, I had to do "the dance" (you know the steps!) complete with sucking in and squirming to help get them on. As you know by now, that was the turning point that inspired me to make some real changes. I told myself there was no way I was going to buy a size 38 inch waist pants when most of my adult life I had been wearing a size 34. It was traumatic enough going from a 34 inch waist to a 36, and I was determined that trend was going to stop.

Measure your progress by how your clothes fit. Are they loose or too tight? Candidly, I hadn't been on a scale in years and had no idea how bad the problem truly was based on the numbers. Being aware of how my clothes fit gave me a good indication that I needed to take action right away. Now that I've lost the weight and have been able to maintain my current weight of 155 lbs., I can tell you without a doubt, I feel a tremendous sense of accomplishment when I wear my 31 inch waist pants. I'm not talking about having just one or two pairs in that size, but every pair of pants in my closet now have a 31 inch waist. In fact, I even have two pairs of 30's. OK, they're labeled "relaxed fit," but 30's are 30's nevertheless, right?

I also feel good wearing either a small or medium shirt when I previously needed a large. This doesn't give me quite the same level of satisfaction as my waist size because I personally think today's small is yesterday's medium. The whole population is getting so overweight, I believe the manufacturers have simply adjusted the clothing sizes upward to accommodate this trend. Admittedly, you may feel better because you can now wear a small instead of a medium. I know I sure do. Give yourself a pat on the back if you're wearing a smaller size because you've lost inches. Just be aware that you could be wearing the smaller size simply because manufacturers are modifying the sizes to fit our "growing" population.

Moving beyond the scale and your clothes, why not determine your body fat percentage. Historically, body fat percentage is a little more difficult to measure because the devices to measure it are not as readily available to purchase. If you've done any scale shopping lately, many of the recent models are including the body fat percentage feature in the scale itself. This metric can be quite sobering as the name implies. When my weight peaked, my body fat was in the mid 30% range. This meant that about 1/3 of my body weight was made up of fat. I know, gross, isn't it. Now that I'm down to 155 pounds and have built solid lean muscle, my body fat is about 13%. That percentage drop is a significant motivator to keep me going in an effort to maintain my goal weight and body composition.

Some people try to lose weight by following the starvation approach. They severely cut down on their daily calorie consumption thinking that it will speed up their weight loss. However, this depravation approach simply puts the body into starvation mode which can never be sustained. If they're monitoring their body fat percentage, they'll see that they're losing muscle mass. You want to be building muscle, not losing it, as you strive to achieve a sustainable, healthy lifestyle.

As you measure progress toward your weight loss and fitness goal, use all of the tools available to indicate your progress: the scale, the way your clothes fit, and your body fat percentage just to name a few. You'll begin to see the bigger picture of how you're doing. The scale isn't the only measure of success; it's just one of many tools that can help you succeed in your weight loss and fitness efforts.

You and the Mirror

1. Go through your closet and find items of clothing that used to fit that currently do not. Take them out and hang them somewhere so that you can see them. List below the items you found and their sizes:

   Item_____ Size_____

   Item_____ Size_____

   Item_____ Size_____

2. Research body composition scales, which include weight, body fat %, and body composition, on the Internet and record the manufacturer and price below:

   Manufacturer_____ Price_____

   Manufacturer_____ Price_____

   Manufacturer_____ Price_____

   Manufacturer_____ Price_____

   Consider purchasing a body composition scale. If you don't think you can afford it today, add it to your fitness budget for a future purchase.

Ah Ha #19: Take Lots of Pictures; They Don't Lie

We've all seen the late night infomercials that show the before and after pictures of a person losing a tremendous amount of weight and miraculously and effortlessly getting the ripped abs. This is certainly the extreme and, in fact, the tiny print at the bottom of the TV screen confirms this. However, I've found that looking at old pictures can actually be motivating.

If you're at the point where you're fed up with your weight like I was and you're committed to becoming healthy, I strongly encourage you to take some photographs of yourself. This is the one thing that I regret not doing enough of prior to starting my weight loss journey. Fortunately, I had a few loose photos illustrating my old body type that I could use to remind myself that I never want to look like that again.

As you look at your current pictures, be honest and say to yourself, "I never want to go back to that." This visual reminder can motivate you to stick with your plan. When you are heavier, you most likely shy away from the camera. As you begin to lose weight and get comfortable with your own fitness and nutrition regime, you'll be surprised how often you'll want your picture taken. You may even be elbowing others out of the frame so that you can be front and center. Once you take that picture, that image is trapped in time. It will always be there. Pictures don't lie.

I was so disgusted by one picture, the one with me in the ocean on my Web site, that when I first got it developed, I physically threw it away. I couldn't stand to look at it. It showed me at my heaviest. It was horrible. However, I decided to use it as my "before" picture on the cover of this book. Since I no longer had the print, I had to take the negative to the local Ritz camera so that they could make me another one.

Don't shy away from pictures. If you're just starting out in your journey, take lots of them. Stage some of the shots so that you can do real *before and after*s in the same clothes with the same backdrop. You will be so incredibly proud of yourself when you reach your goals and display those old flabby clothes that used to be tight on you, with the same backdrop. Those are results that can never be taken away.

Ah Ha #19: Take Lots of Pictures; They Don't Lie

You and the Mirror

1. Review some old pictures and find one that is just awful and you're embarrassed to look at. Put it up on the fridge for motivation and tape a copy in the space below:

2. Take a "before" picture using a backdrop that will be there in a few months. You should wear somewhat revealing clothing to get the full effect of your current body condition. Plan to take an "after" picture on your pre-selected goal date wearing the same clothes with the same backdrop. Tape both pictures below:

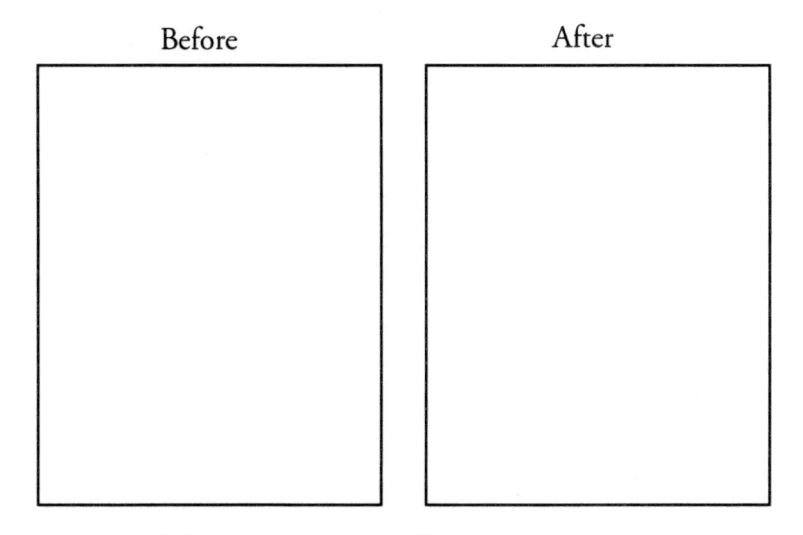

Before   After

Ah Ha #20: Never Too Late to Start

No matter what exercise you choose, whether it's walking, jogging, cycling, swimming or participating in a group fitness class, remember—it's never too late to start. Some folks get into a rut and say things such as, *"Well, I've had this body type for the last 20 years. What's going to change now?"* If you're not currently following an exercise and nutrition program, the time to start is now.

While I was creating JumpSnap, I was inspired by the wide age range of people who were interested in the product and universally excited about trying it. I gained a great deal of satisfaction knowing that it wouldn't be the type of product that people would grow out of. This broad market appeal is what ultimately gave me the confidence to press on to develop it.

One of my favorite success stories that's proof positive you're never too old to start features Jerry, a 68-year-old man who was an older participant in a 50-person focus group. The focus group participants used JumpSnap three days a week. At the end of the 12-week session, Jerry had lost 30 lbs. overall and over 9 inches off his waist. All he did was JumpSnap three days a week for 12 weeks and learned about nutrition in the process. He wasn't even big all over, but he carried it in the most dangerous part of the body, the midsection. To his credit, he was 68 years old and made the change when he just as easily could have accepted his overweight body.

Jerry's story really proves a point that no matter where you are in life, regardless of age, you have the ability to change. All that is required is that you determine that you want to change and then you follow through to make the change happen. To me, it was really inspirational that, at Jerry's age, he wanted to take control, make the change, and ultimately lost the weight (especially in the most dangerous area of his body, his midsection).

Not only do people who exercise regularly and eat healthy lose weight and improve their fitness level, they also tend to look younger than they did in their "before" pictures. Many of the hit reality shows that deal with obesity are proving this point time and time again. For those participants who are severely over weight, I'm amazed by how much younger they look after they lose the weight. The weight loss always boosts their confidence and self esteem, and all of this transformation occurs because of their steadfast commitment to exercise and nutrition, and not because of plastic surgery, liposuction, or flush diets.

I've heard so many stories of people who had pretty much given up because they hadn't found an exercise or weight loss program that worked for them. My advice is to keep pushing on, take advantage of some of the basics I learned along the way and recognize that you're never too old to start. You absolutely can change your body type and look a little younger in the process.

You and the Mirror

1. Find healthy adults in the following age groups and ask what they do for exercise and how many times they do this activity per week:

AGE RANGE	Exercise Activity/# of times a week
20-30 year old	_____
31-40 year old	_____
41-50 year old	_____
51-60 year old	_____
61-70 year old	_____
Over 70	_____

2. What exercise activity do you do now and how often do you do it?

   _____

3. What exercise activities are you not currently doing that you would like to start doing?

4. What type of exercise activity do you think you'll be doing when you're 70 years old?

Ah Ha #21: Anything Worth Having Takes Hard Work and Commitment

Pardon the preaching, but we all need a little reality check once in a while. Whether we're talking about health and fitness, our jobs or our relationships, any meaningful achievement requires hard work.

I always found it odd that I was successful in my career and would do whatever it took to get ahead at the office. Yet, I would slough off when it came to exercise. Why is it that we can be so efficient in the office or around the house when it's for someone else, but when it's for ourselves, we don't give it the same level of attention? Hey, I'm no Dr. Phil, but I want to challenge you to put yourself first when it comes to health and fitness.

Let me be clear here. I'm not saying that you should under perform at work because you need to excel in your personal life. Just give your personal goals the same level of professionalism you likely take for granted at work, and I bet you'll be pleased with the results.

Be honest with yourself when it comes to expectations and commitment. You would never tell a client you can do something by tomorrow close of business if, in fact, you knew it was going to take two weeks to accomplish. Apply that same approach to your own fitness goals, and you'll be pleasantly surprised with the results.

If you're not currently exercising at all, start by committing to three days per week and build from there. If you set a course for exercising on Monday, Wednesday, and Friday and a business or family function pops up on a Wednesday, don't freak out and scrap your entire workout. Take a deep breath and consider any number of logical alternatives. If you typically work out in the evening, how about getting up a little earlier that day so that you can work out in the morning? Or perhaps change your exercise schedule for the week to Monday, Tuesday and Thursday?

I know this sounds so basic and trivial, but from my personal experience, I know how easy it is to get derailed by one simple interruption. From there, negative rationalizations and excuses that we all face take over, and the next thing you know it's been two weeks and you haven't broken a sweat. Don't accept that mental manipulation. Stay committed to yourself.

If losing weight and staying fit were easy, we'd all be buff and at our ideal weight. It requires hard work and commitment to achieve your goal, but the payoff is well worth it, and in this case, it's life saving.

Ah Ha #21: Anything Worth Having Takes Hard Work and Commitment

You and the Mirror

1. Fill in the blanks and sign and date the following commitment:

I realize that to achieve my fitness and weight loss goals I need to work hard and stay steadfast in my commitment to achieving them. I realize that I am solely responsible for achieving my goals and that nobody else can do it for me.

I promise to *(fill in your exercise program—for example, ride a bicycle)* _____ on *(insert days of the week—for example, on Monday, Wednesday, and Friday)* _____ _____ for *(insert amount of time for your workout, for example, for 45 minutes)* _____.

Signature _____ Date _____

2. When was the last time you skipped a workout?

    What was your reason for doing so?

    What did you do to make up for it?

Ah Ha #22: The Dreaded Annual Physical

Most of us grew up getting an annual physical for school, only because we had to. We got the required vaccines and notches on the chart for height and weight. After high school, however, many of us stopped going to the doctor for regular check ups. We tended to go to the doctor only if we were sick in search of antibiotics or medical relief as opposed to preventative care.

If you're a healthy 20 something, you might be able to get away with skipping the annual exam. The problem is, however, many of us fail to have an annual physical when we probably should have one. Now I'm not certain if there is a medically recommended age whereby you should receive an annual physical, but I encourage you, if it's been awhile, to pick up the phone right now and make an appointment. You're probably OK, but why risk it. Many times if physical problems are detected early, something can be done about them with little discomfort or long-term consequences. An annual exam also gives you the chance to talk with your doctor about preventative care.

Making an appointment for an annual physical is another badge of honor that demonstrates you are taking ownership of your health. Be proud of the fact that you care enough about yourself to block off one hour each year from your busy life to get a check-up. Another benefit is that you can begin to build some historical background on the key health metrics to gage how well you're doing. In my case, I know that every summer is my time to get my physical. Because I

Ah Ha #22: The Dreaded Annual Physical

know I will be weighed at that appointment, there is a subtle pressure to be in good shape.

When at the doctor's office, don't be afraid to talk about a healthy lifestyle or even use him or her as a sounding board to learn about health and nutrition. Prior to my weight loss, my doctor was very helpful because he would give me honest answers about diet supplements or fad diets. Here is a chart of my results for the past few years.

Year	Weight	Cholesterol	HDL (the good one)	LDL (the bad one)	Triglycerides
2002	189	151	38	91	112
2003	190	170	52	82	179
2004	205	I was too embarrassed to go			
2005	178	163	50	79	170
2006	161	146	51	77	88
2007	155	146	52	80	68

Seeing the numbers makes you strive toward a healthy lifestyle. If you can see them, you can do something about them. If the numbers are not what you want them to be, you can talk with your doctor about taking corrective action to get on the right track. However, if you never go to the doctor and don't have these numbers, you're just shooting in the dark. As in Ah Ha #17, you can't reach your goal tomorrow if you don't know where you are today.

If you don't want to go to the doctor for an annual physical for selfish reasons or because you're too embarrassed, do it for our financially burdened health care system. Prevention is always the better route than waiting till you have a serious health issue and then having to undergo expensive treatments. Getting your medical scorecard updated each year is an easy way to raise awareness for any irregular test results. It's always cheaper to catch something on the front end as opposed to letting it go until it's a significant problem.

Make the annual pilgrimage to the doctor. Take good care of your body. It's the only one you're ever going to have.

The Ah Ha's of Weight Loss

You and the Mirror

1. When was the last time you had an annual physical? _____

2. When is your next annual physical scheduled?
   _____

3. Fill in your medical scorecard with the key numbers from your previous visits (however many years you have available) and continue to add to the chart through the years. (You may need to contact your doctor's office and get the numbers from your records.)

Year	Weight	Cholesterol	HDL (the good one)	LDL (the bad one)	Triglycerides

4. What are the numbers telling you? What are you doing right? What can you do better?

Ah Ha #23: If You Really Love Them, Be Honest

As the adage goes, honesty is the best policy. Yep, even when it comes to weight loss and fitness. Since this Ah Ha deals with the most precious people in our lives—our family and friends—it can be a sensitive one.

We are taught to love people unconditionally. That means that no matter how they look or what they do, we're supposed to love and support them. And that's true. In my opinion, however, part of loving them is being honest with them. We may think we're protecting them and "loving" them by keeping them from "seeing" the truth when in fact we're doing the opposite. In the long run, we're actually hurting them.

If a family member or close friend is searching for honest feedback, you should give it to them. Just be careful about how you deliver the message. Avoid being harshly critical, condescending, or intentionally hurtful. Show your love by delivering the message in a very caring and supportive way.

As we look at our epidemic of obesity and more specifically childhood obesity, I'm amazed by whom we are holding responsible. Should we really be blaming 7-, 8- and 9-year olds for being overweight? It's the people who I hope love them the most who are also slowly killing them—their parents. This Ah Ha should make you take a step back, look in the mirror and say, "I need to be honest." Instead of looking around to find someone else to blame, look very closely and ask, "What is my true responsibility to myself and others?"

Sometimes you need to be very upfront and open and actually ask people for their honest feedback and support. This reaching out to others is powerful because it opens the door and lays the groundwork for how you want to be supported.

In my pursuit towards a more active lifestyle, I proactively reached out to my wife for support. I first asked her to gently remind me from time to time about my goals. I asked her to join me in eating more healthy options, even though she didn't need to lose weight. I asked her to give me a friendly nudge if I wasn't doing the workouts when I said I was going to. I allowed her to be part of my own success cheerleading squad by telling her what I wanted to achieve, which enabled her to keep me honest. Voicing and communicating that "I'm putting you on notice that I'm taking on these challenges. I want to do this and may reach a point where I need a friendly reminder." That's how somebody can really help you, but you need to be proactive to make it happen.

How do you open the door to provide honest feedback and support to others? As you are more and more successful in your own health and fitness transformation, you'll begin to serve as a role model. People will start looking to you for feedback on how they can also improve their lives.

When you provide feedback, make sure you're delivering the right messages at the right time, but more importantly focus on the way you deliver your messages (how you say it more so than what you say). Try not to hurt their feelings or damage their self-esteem. Family members and friends who know you really care about them will be grateful, especially in the long-term, if you're able to be honest and let them know that you care. They'll realize that you want to be there as part of their support system to enable them to reach their goals and live a longer and more vibrant life.

Ah Ha #23: If You Really Love Them, Be Honest

You and the Mirror

1. Write below the script you will use to ask a family member or close friend to support you in your journey toward a healthier and more active lifestyle:

2. Now, look in the mirror and practice reading your script aloud. Note your body language and facial expressions as you deliver your message to yourself.

    What do you like about your delivery?

    What do you need to change?

3. If you've already achieved your goal weight, think about the people closest to you who could benefit from your success. Write down three people whom you think you can impact towards leading a more healthy life.

    _____

    _____

    _____

Ah Ha #24: "Overnight Success" — Only In Hollywood

Professional athletes practice their sport for years before they make it to the pros. Young pop stars probably have been practicing and performing since they were toddlers before they hit the big time. CEOs of some of the most successful companies and even self-made entrepreneurs didn't achieve their level of success overnight. Their success was many years in the making. When a new up-and-coming singer or actor hits the scene, it creates a buzz. Since we had never heard of them before, we assume they got lucky with a big break. We are unaware of the long arduous road they have taken as they worked their way to the top.

The problem with all of these alleged overnight success stories is that they are romanticized by the media to sell newspapers, magazines, concert tickets, or movie tickets. They can certainly be very inspiring, but take them with a grain of salt. Consider how long it actually took them to translate their years and even decades of hard work into a success.

When people hear about the success of JumpSnap, for the most part they have no idea what I have had to do to make it a success. Why is that? Well, since I haven't been in the fitness business or product marketing business before, I had no name recognition. The real story is that it took me almost a decade to take JumpSnap from a concept in my head to a final sellable product. Now granted,

Ah Ha #24: "Overnight Success" — Only In Hollywood

there were many years of grave doubt and time spent working for someone else that slowed down progress, but it still took a good bit of time to get it rolling. Now that my product and I are getting to be a little more well-known, even my story could be sensationalized as an overnight success.

Another great success story involves my good friend, Mike Walden. (I referenced Mike in the Acknowledgement because we've been best friends since 7th grade, and he actually helped me start my business.) Following college graduation, Mike and I competed in several triathlons and ran a marathon together. Just like my situation, Mike allowed the challenges of every day life to get in the way of living a healthy lifestyle. As a result, he also put on a few extra unwanted pounds. Over the years Mike had talked about completing one of the most grueling challenges in sport, The Iron Man race (2.5 mile swim, 112 mile bike, 26.2 mile run). He thanks me, to some extent, for inspiring him to take on the challenge. As he tells the story, his "enough is enough" moment came when I offered him my fat pants. After all, what are friends for? Immediately, Mike dusted off his 10-year-old dream, and began training. After two years of countless hours in the pool, on the bike and on the road, Mike successfully completed the Madison Iron Man. He not only achieved his goal of completing it, but he posted an unbelievable time of 11 hours and 30 minutes to finish in the top 15% of the entire field, including the pros. Throughout his journey, he lost 35 lbs. and gained an appreciation for the impact that pursuing a healthy lifestyle has made on every facet of his life. Congrats again, Waldo. Awesome job!

Why am I talking about all this? Because I want you to be realistic about your own transformation. It takes time, so don't get frustrated when it's not happening overnight when you think it should. If you let the frustration get the best of you, you may get discouraged and end up quitting all together. The only people who want that to happen are the people who are developing and promoting the next great diet plan or pill, so that you'll be suckered into buying them.

Like most people, it took me years to add on the weight. Why would I be so unrealistic to think it would come off in just a few short weeks? Sure, I'd love to tell people that I lost the weight in two weeks, like promoters of the magic pills claim, but that's just absurd. You need to allow your new habits and disciplines to take effect. That certainly takes time.

If you look at the real history behind any business, product, service, virtually any success story, you'll discover that it took years if not decades to get it to the point where the public sees it as an overnight success. Right or wrong, realize that to get there required a lot of work, patience, and fortitude. If success were easy, everybody would be famous.

Ah Ha #24: "Overnight Success" — Only In Hollywood

You and the Mirror

1. Write below your description of what success would look like as it relates to your weight loss and fitness goals.

2. "You can't achieve success unless you know what it is." Agree or disagree with this statement and explain the reasons for your choice.

Ah Ha #25: Obesity Facts — You Can Make A Difference!

So what's the payoff for making a commitment to leading a healthy lifestyle? If you follow good nutritional guidelines, exercise regularly and set realistic and achievable goals, the payoff will be evident in many facets of your life. By living a healthy lifestyle you will become a positive role model to your family, friends and all those who surround you, whether you realize it or not.

The other payoff is that you can, even in a small way, help combat the obesity epidemic that is costing a staggering $100 billion/year just to treat obesity-related illnesses. According to the Center for Disease Control, obesity is the #1 cause for health-related issues, such as the early onset of Type-2 diabetes and heart-related diseases.

Imagine what we can do one person at a time, one family at a time, one neighborhood at a time, and one community at a time by taking a look at ourselves and making the commitment to take better care of ourselves—and then helping and supporting each other to make these commitments a reality. Imagine the preventive impact that having a healthier population would have on the amount of money spent on treating obesity-related illnesses, a number that has grown exponentially year over year. It's mind-blowing, when you think about that. Over $100 billion is spent annually on hard medical costs on dealing with the illness itself (medical treatment of obesity and obesity-related illnesses), not to mention the soft costs of absenteeism and decreased productivity and how they affect the economy.

Obesity is one of those conditions that we can do something about. Weight loss reality shows prove this time and time again. Contestants often start the show with a series of ailments, and once they get their weight into check, those ailments either go away completely or are drastically reduced. If that doesn't illustrate the power resulting from getting your health and fitness in line, I don't know what does. It's unbelievable—and commendable.

We must look to ourselves for the solution to the obesity epidemic because we can make a difference. We will benefit by living a healthier lifestyle with more confidence and exuberance and by being able to do all the things we've always wanted to do. What a wonderful way to help our economy by removing this pressure that we're all placing on the overall system.

If we look at ourselves and close-knit group of family and friends, we can start chipping away at the obesity problem. Let's look to solve the nationwide epidemic by looking in our own homes first. Thank you for sharing your time with me and committing to healthy living. I wish you huge success in your personal journey and hope these Ah Ha's lend support towards achieving your goals.

You and the Mirror

1. Write below what you will do in your own home to fight the obesity problem.

2. What can you do in your neighborhood and community to combat the obesity problem?

3. List below the people you will enlist to help you fight the obesity problem.

My Ah Ha's Journal to Healthy Living

About the Author

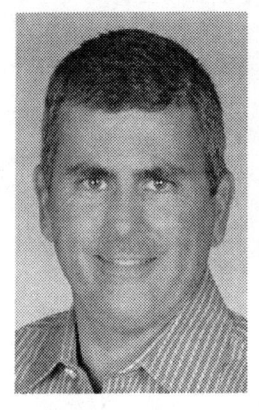

Brad LaTour has taken an unusual path to share his personal story of weight loss, reinvention and taking on the role of being a healthy living advocate. A relative newcomer to the fitness business, Brad's journey began when he invented **JumpSnap**. As the weight began coming off, it peaked his interest to learn more about the fundamentals of leveraging exercise and nutrition to lose weight and keep it off. His advice cuts through the clutter with the simplicity of his message and how easily it can be integrated into our busy lives. This book is a repository for all the **'Ah Ha'** moments Brad had along his journey, and now he can share those moments with others to help them on their quest to live healthy lives.

Brad's greatest inspiration comes from the constant flow of success stories he receives on a daily basis. It provides further validation that he has made the right choice to turn his passion into a full time job and commitment.

In addition to selling JumpSnap worldwide, Brad has created a health and wellness portal called **JumpSnap Nation**. It provides members with a forum to share their stories, seek advice from the stable of JSN fitness and nutrition experts, and focus on healthy living. His passion for helping others also led him to create **My Fitness 1st**, a foundation to help eliminate childhood obesity.

www.jumpsnap.com
www.jumpsnapnation.com
www.myfitness1st.org

The *Ah Ha's* of *Weight Loss*

- ✔ Have you ever tried a diet and failed?
- ✔ Have you ever told yourself this is going to be the year you will lose weight and get healthy?
- ✔ Have you ever started exercising but gave up because you didn't see immediate results?
- ✔ Have you wanted to believe there is a pill to solve your weight problems?

If you shook your head 'yes' to any of these or are still nodding because you answered 'yes' to all of them, you are not alone. There is a good chance you are probably a lot like the author, Brad LaTour, who struggled for years to get a handle on his weight gain.

There is something different about this book. Unlike the next great weight loss cure, diet, pill, lotion, potion or surgery, this book delivers some practical answers. Finally, you will hear from someone who you can identify with because he's been there. You will enjoy his refreshingly honest approach about how to put yourself on a path toward healthy living. And more importantly, it will give you the confidence of knowing that implementing several small changes is truly the only way to lose weight and keep it off.

It's time to let go of the failed attempts in the past and use LaTour's story and tools to finally treat yourself to the healthy body you've always envisioned.